ADVANCE PRAISE

"I was lucky enough to get my hands on Love what you Wear before anyone else. After 3 chapters, I was torn between finishing the book and hiring Alexandra immediately. It became so clear that there was a lot to know about style and I didn't know enough. Just the few tidbits she shared about color made it so clear why even though my outfits looked fashionable, they didn't look good or feel good on me. It's so much more than just fashion. It's about showing up authentically and consciously choosing to look good as me, not the current fad or trend. Thank you Alexandra for your wisdom and I can't wait for our time together!"

–Alisabeth Ann Shelman

"This is a must own book for the woman who lives in multiple locations. Living in San Francisco and NYC requires a varied wardrobe - but who wants to lug around their entire wardrobe? The organizational tips in *Love What You Wear* are invaluable when it comes to looking your best in every situation. You don't need a Wall Street suit in Silicon Valley or a hoodie for NYC."

–Lilli Balfour

T0124446

"*Love What You Wear* is a charming yet comprehensive guide through a women's ongoing issue of what to wear, not just in multiple homes, even for those with one closet. Because of her lifelong 'luxury-nomadic' lifestyle, Ms. Greenawalt offers incredibly insightful yet simple solutions on why we have a closet packed with clothes we don't wear, how to overcome buying the wrong things, and finally dress with style and confidence, becoming of our body and skin tone. Whether you're in multiple locations or the one city you call home, her advice helps lift the stress of what to wear and makes dressing up fun again. Thank you Alexandra! "

–Cristen Chambers
of Portland, Oregon, Oysterville, Washington,
and Miami, Florida

"In her previous publications, Alexandra Suzanne Greenawalt has always had an extraordinarily intuitive and almost visceral comprehension of style – an understanding that seems almost to live at the cellular level. No wonder her style advice is couched in almost physiological terms. In her new book, she writes of 'detoxing' your wardrobe, and avoiding 'shopping hangovers.' She isn't just a stylist – she's a style physician!"

–Mark Gauthier

"Alexandra has done it again. This book is full of common sense advice delivered by a Pro who really knows her stuff. As a professional organizer, I can attest to the methods Alexandra recommends in the DETOX section of LWYW. Being able to find things in your closet is the first step to looking and feeling great. This is just the starting point. This book walks you through all the steps for realizing your own personal (comfortable) style, no matter how many homes you own!"

–Anne Garrymore, AnneGarrymore.com

"*Love What You Wear* is a style must-read. I appreciate that Alexandra Suzanne Greenawalt shares many of her fashion secrets in a helpful, often hilarious manner. I actually paused reading a couple of chapters in because I couldn't help but "detox" my closet immediately! Thanks to this book, I feel like I'm on the road toward becoming a fashionista."

–Sandi Brager

"As a one-domicile woman who occasionally travels, I found Alexandra's book full of information to help me assess my wardrobe, weed it and make changes that will help me dress better and feel better about how I look at home or away."

–Vicky Cohen

"I have to say that this book is NOT about only those of us who have two or even three houses and consequent closets to manage. I have down sized and live in a guest house on our big property. Even with my shrinking closets of what I have always known, half of that space is full of clothes that are waiting for me to become 60 again...I am now in my 70'S. Give it up! I love this book!"

–Linda Mornell

"Having read and enjoyed Alexandra's previous book, "Vetted By A Stylist" I was super excited when she offered me a sneak peek at *Love What You Wear*. My aha moment came in chapter 3. Although I reside in New York City, I'm fortunate enough to have a weekend home on the north fork of Long Island. Lovely, full of farmland and vineyards, for years I've shuttled my wardrobe back and forth between there and the city. But I never felt comfortable in my city clothes, out there. And, thanks to Alexandra, now I know why: I'm a chameleon trying to be a uniform dresser (see page 19)! My thought had always been "I haven't changed, why should my clothes?" Alexandra made me realize that, mastering your style (in my case, having multiple wardrobes) wasn't about being self-indulgent or frivolous: it was about streamlining my life so that I was comfortable enough in my own skin, that I could be myself wherever I was. *Love What You Wear* teaches you how to keep from being a slave to your wardrobe – so that you can focus on what's really important! Thanks, Alexandra!"

–Dawn Vicknair, actress

"A style journal from a creative nomadic stylist who can better your wardrobe with the certainty you have what you love in every closet in your multi-homes, hotels, air-streamers or yachts!"

–Juel Bedford

"Alexandra has such a timeless, chic sense of style which is definitely conveyed in her latest book, *Love What You Wear*. After reading her book, I am completely motivated to "detox" my wardrobe, which will undoubtedly give me a fresh perspective on my personal style. While our second home is in the mountains, far from the sharp eye of the fashion police, we do quite a bit of traveling. I am thrilled I was given the opportunity to read her book before our spring trip to Europe, as I will be using her extremely helpful style and packing tips. I am determined not to overpack, yet with Alexandra's help, I will make every effort to look stylish in every port. I recommend this book to anyone who needs a little guidance in finding their personal flair, multiple homes or not!"

–Julie Ann Ulcickas

OTHER BOOKS BY
ALEXANDRA SUZANNE GREENAWALT:

Secrets of a Fashion Stylist

Vetted by a Stylist

LOVE WHAT YOU WEAR

LOVE WHAT YOU WEAR

Mastering Your Style in Multiple Homes

ALEXANDRA SUZANNE GREENAWALT

NEW YORK

LONDON • NASHVILLE • MELBOURNE • VANCOUVER

LOVE WHAT YOU WEAR

Mastering Your Style in Multiple Homes

© 2018 Alexandra Suzanne Greenawalt

All rights reserved. No portion of this book may be reproduced, stored in a retrieval system, or transmitted in any form or by any means—electronic, mechanical, photocopy, recording, scanning, or other—except for brief quotations in critical reviews or articles, without the prior written permission of the publisher.

Published in New York, New York, by Morgan James Publishing in partnership with Difference Press. Morgan James is a trademark of Morgan James, LLC. www.MorganJamesPublishing.com

The Morgan James Speakers Group can bring authors to your live event. For more information or to book an event visit The Morgan James Speakers Group at www.TheMorganJamesSpeakersGroup.com.

ISBN 9781683506331 paperback
ISBN 9781683506348 eBook
Library of Congress Control Number: 2017909664

Cover and Interior Design by:
Chris Treccani
www.3dogcreative.net

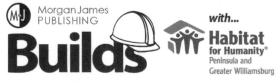

In an effort to support local communities, raise awareness and funds, Morgan James Publishing donates a percentage of all book sales for the life of each book to Habitat for Humanity Peninsula and Greater Williamsburg.

Get involved today! Visit
www.MorganJamesBuilds.com

DEDICATION

For my Grandfather who inspired me to be an entrepreneur
+
For my Grandmother who inspired me with her infinite style

TABLE OF CONTENTS

FOREWORD

Through my decades of environmental work, I've developed a philosophy of minimalism and mindfulness. I embrace this philosophy in all aspects of my life, especially when it comes to material consumption and finding ways to enjoy fashion while streamlining my purchases.

Although I try to buy less and minimize my carbon footprint, I travel very often for my work and need to have a dynamic wardrobe to suit varying weather and climate conditions as well as cultural factors including formal dress and cover-up, excursions and touring, speaking engagements and professional dress for work.

I've also been booked on back-to-back flights in different time-zones, from cold and damp to hot and humid temperatures, and I've dealt with the challenge of squeezing outfit options and items I "might wear" into a carry-on luggage bag to avoid checking it at airports. All this, along with lists of what are my essentials for packing are well-addressed in Alexandra Greenawalt's book *Love What You Wear*.

Alexandra's book helps readers to lessen the pressure of having too many nonessentials and provides thoughtful and at times humorous insight to what is relevant to any woman who is on the go and wants to pack wisely while upholding her personal sense of style.

Alexandra spent her formative years living between her multiple family homes, identifying her must-pack pieces and coming up with fun and creative ways to make the most of her travel essentials. In this spirit, *Love What You Wear* helps you identify which questions to ask yourself while packing, and provides tips for dressing up and dressing down your wardrobe.

The knowledge Alexandra shares in the following pages has the potential to make your life easier. She'll guide you in selecting your staple items, adjusting your buying patterns to make smarter purchases, streamlining your wardrobe, and curating your style. Alexandra has an engaging voice and her often humorous stories from her days as a stylist and a fashion organizer allow you to consider ways to streamline your own style so that it works for your body type, skin tone, eye color, et cetera.

Love What You Wear teaches you how to creatively and critically express your personal values through your clothing while empowering you to feel confident, powerful and prepared for anything. Thank you Alexandra for this timely book for the modern traveler and working woman.

–Susan Rockefeller
Founder and Editor-in-Chief musingsmag.com

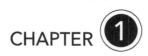

EXPLODING CLOSETS AND NOTHING TO WEAR

Have you ever gotten home from the grocery store with $100 dollars worth of groceries but then realized you don't have the right ingredients to make a meal?

You shopped based on what inspired you but without any real plan of what you were going to make.

You have the meat but not the seasonings or the veggies.

You have fantastic artisan truffles, but you're not sure what to do with them.

This is also exactly what happens to women and shopping.

They see a fabulous piece, have to have it and purchase it but with no real understanding or plan of what to wear it with.

And then it sits in the closet unworn and lonely, never taken for a walk outside.

So you go back to the department store, spend more money, maybe with a personal shopper, and find more fabulous statement worthy pieces but with no mates.

And you have contacts with the sales girls at all the boutiques, and you shop there with their 'help'.

You shop and shop, yet you never feel you have anything to wear that feels like you.

And this cycle repeats itself.

And soon your many closets are bursting with items that you aren't wearing.

This is one of the reasons most women only wear 20% of their closets.

You're bringing more items into your houses and closets and not much are going out.

How can you donate an item that you spent hundreds of dollars on that still has the tags on?

It feels wasteful you say.

It feels like you're admitting failure.

If you're not in the habit of pruning and editing out pieces that you haven't worn, your closet doesn't get any more manageable with time.

Just worse.

Until you reach a breaking point.

You may be at that breaking point now.

Anne, beautiful in her 40s, lives on Park Avenue near the Guggenheim Museum and spends weekends during the winter in her home in Palm Beach with her husband. In the summer they weekend at their house in the Hamptons. They are newly married. Anne works in the healing industry and has worked very hard to build her expanding practice. Her husband is also very successful. They are social but mainly prefer to hang out at home. They do attend black tie events during the year and it's usually because of accepting awards. Anne is well aware of the social norms in the scene and how most women dress. She is not interested in looking like all the other women; she wants to look elegant, chic, down to earth, and in control. She is also well aware that the circle they frequent in Palm Beach at the private clubs is a whole different monster, style-wise. Her husband likes to get involved in her clothing and often buys her outfits from Ralph Lauren, but Anne doesn't feel good about her wardrobe or her style. She just grabs her favorite jeans and t-shirt. She jokes that in her fancy NYC building, the way she dresses, she is mistaken for staff.

She is equally paralyzed about wearing the items in her closet whether they're dressy or casual. Her closets are filled with expensive clothing and accessories, most of which don't get worn. She has lots of items that are black but also lots of pieces with hardware, zippers, embellishments, prints, basically strong pieces. She wears about 10% of her closet, mostly her jeans and white t-shirts. She has lots of 'orphan pieces that have no mates' but have lots of personality. Still, Anne thinks that somewhere in her closet there are mates, but she just doesn't know them. When she is in Palm Beach she often goes to wear an outfit and then realizes that the perfect purse for the outfit is at a different home, and she's not sure which one. And none of the purses she has at this house work with this outfit. She's not one to stress about 'style' things because she has much more important stuff in her life, but these 'tiny' challenges do throw a cog in her wheel. She finds herself paralyzed and not sure what to wear. She knows women can be gossipy about what people wear to what event.

In the Hamptons they are more casual, but she has things in her closet there that she shuttled from other homes because they weren't getting worn. But they still aren't getting worn in the Hamptons either.

This is where I come in. I've helped women with multiple homes achieve style success. And you don't need to change yourself. You don't need a perfect body. You don't need more or less stuff; you just need the RIGHT amount of stuff for your life and homes.

In this book, you're going to learn the exact styling process I use with my private clients and how you can create a system that works for you and your current lifestyle. For best results, make sure to download the free workbook, which you can download at AlexandraStylist.com/workbook, as I'll be referring to it throughout the following pages.

The style prescription process includes four major steps:

~ DEFINE
~ DETOX
~ SHOP
~ STYLE

Ready? Great, let's get rolling.

CHAPTER 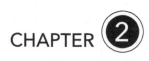 2

WHY I DO THIS WORK

"look fabulous
be legendary
appear complex
act easy
radiate presence
travel light
seem a dream
prove real"
- Talbot's ad from the late 90's

As a child of divorce in Northern California at the tender age of 5, I understood deeply what it meant to live in multiple homes and be semi-nomadic. My father moved onto his 50-foot sailboat where I also spent time. I learned to adapt, like heating up my clothing in the morning by placing it on the heater and making due with a tiny closet. When my father moved into a condo, I shared my room with my brother and had to cope with no dresser. Later as a teenager, I was shuttled between two homes- at mom and dad's I was always saying, "Where is my favorite sweater?" I was constantly losing things and feeling discombobulated about what I was going to wear. And style was VERY important to me. I felt that the secret to being a cool kid in school was rad outfits. I was a big Madonna fan so playing dress-up after school was a highlight of my childhood.

When I went away to boarding school on the east coast at age 14 things got even more complicated stuff-wise with mom's house and dad's house, boarding school, and then on top of it, I usually went to sleep away summer camp in places like Oxford, England; New Hampshire; and Paris. I'm not complaining. I was really lucky and very fortunate. But I knew the importance of packing and felt very frustrated about how to have what I needed to wear when I needed it.

Also, having very dressy grandparents who lived in the preppy world, was a lesson in how to dress appropriately based on your environment. I learned very early on that what one wears in Northern California is very different from Hobe Sound, Florida. At age 12 we went on safari with my mother and brother and a whole wardrobe so different from California was needed to cope with the dust and wildlife lifestyle. I realized that it was really important to attempt to blend in, so I enjoyed buying outfits there to wear in Kenya.

I started shopping accordingly to be able to move in all these different worlds while keeping my style, yet not sticking out too much. I could be a style chameleon and try out different looks depending on where I was in the world. During my prep school days, I found myself ordering from catalogues and being exposed to new designers and styles that were way preppier than what was worn on the West Coast. Laura Ashley was the 'it' designer to get our dresses from and J.Crew for shorts. Today I believe that most women either identify as a chameleon or a uniform dresser. And knowing this will factor in immensely with how you stock each of your homes and suitcases. More about this in future chapters.

My step-grandmother was a huge catalyst in my early style influences, and our trips to Fashion Island are forever etched in my style brain. She was style personified, and she lived in FOUR different houses in FOUR different states. Wow, what a jet setter! GMP (Grandma Pat) was always beautifully turned out, perfectly made up, and with exquisite timeless statement jewelry. The colors and cuts of clothing she wore complemented her skin tone and body perfectly. Her face glowed, and she instinctively knew what colors created that reality. I was in awe of her. I later learned how she made sure she looked fabulous at every house. She would keep basics at each house and then shuttle a van in between them all with her favorite pieces. And she dressed differently based on where she was. Recently she told me if she had wanted to be boring, she would have worn the same thing at every house - but she did NOT. Truly a style icon.

Right out of college I signed up for a course in color and shape analysis with Julie Cunningham Color. I'm not sure how I found out about it, but I was always drawn to style and fashion magazines. I was still lost as to what my career was, but I knew I wanted to know what colors looked good on someone based on skin tone, hair, and eye color. And learning the science of what styles would look good on me, I knew would help me to not feel so frustrated when trying on clothing. In junior high, I was given a clothing allowance and sent off to the mall solo because my mother wasn't into shopping. I was on the small side, so the clothing of the time, baggy 80's pants and shoulder pads, looked ridiculous on me. I already felt like a dork and my clothing wasn't doing me any favors.

So taking this course with Julie Cunningham was life changing! I learned that I was a soft autumn and what kinds of cuts to wear. I learned that black wasn't in my palette! I was in shock because black was one of my main colors and such a big part of my cool identity in college. I came home from the workshop and did a major detox of my closet. It was so easy now to get rid of pieces I wasn't wearing. I finally knew WHY the drop waist black dress didn't look right on me. With my new color knowledge, I started draping my color analysis tester fabrics on anyone who would let me - my grandfather, my mother, my friends, etc. I felt like I had the keys to the puzzle. I later discovered an even more precise system for shape analysis by Bradley Bayou, which included 48 different body types, not 5 types, which made my work all that more powerful. I was excited to help others solve their puzzle. I knew how it felt to feel like a dork or a wallflower, and I didn't want others to feel that way too.

In the 42 years of my life, I've lived in about 34 different places. I know what it means to travel and how challenging it can be to adapt, so isn't it interesting that today I help my clients deal with their multi-layered lives, which include multiple residences.

Today I find myself based in New York City but flirting with other cities. I have yet to settle on a second location of residence but explore sunny parts of the world in the end of summers and during the winter months when the weather is unbearably cold. I generally pick a spot like Los Angeles; Marin County; South Beach, Miami; Crete, Greece; Mallorca, Spain; and Northeast Harbor, Maine. I have welcomed the challenge of how to deal with luggage and what to bring for periods of up to 2-3 months. Being quasi-nomadic has changed the way I pack. Now I pack as if I'm there for 10 days not 2 months, stick to a limited color palette, and create a chameleon capsule wardrobe. I still have fabulous things to wear, but I have way less choices. The minimalism makes the travel more relaxing. I found, by trial, that having too much prevented me from moving around more and exploring. The biggest feat was sticking to 2-3 pairs of shoes. It's brought more ease into my style. To have not more, not less, but just the right amount. And it's fun to pick up new things in town if you need them.

Whether you are living in one large home, 2+ homes, or living out of a suitcase, I have got you covered. You can feel confident, stylish, organized, properly stocked, and sane.

CHAPTER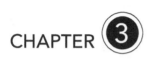

DEFINE

When you have multiple closets and multiple homes there is MORE at stake, since you've already invested so much money in your closets. You may have so much that it overwhelms you. And that's okay because I'm going to walk you through the solutions.

Once you know your style prescription, you can make better choices when editing, shopping, and styling. Loving what you wear is about wiping the slate clean and getting to the root of your style challenges. Rebuilding your wardrobe from the ground up and doing it the conscious way. Making choices carefully, based on a foundation. The foundational work is the most important part of the process because, without this compass, you will continue to be lost. You will continue to purchase items that you aren't sure about and only wear a small portion of what you own. You're going to want to call every sweater in all of your closets your favorite because it looks amazing on you, so that the 'where is my favorite sweater?' conundrum doesn't exist.

Before you can figure out what you need for each closet and home, you need to define your style.

This chapter will explain the first foundational step I take my 1:1 clients through before we do anything else: DEFINE. It's meant to set you up for style success.

The following are all the pieces we need to define:

WHAT LOOKS GOOD ON YOU!?

And I stress YOU because, often when we shop, we fall in love with something on a mannequin or model and don't often think about the relationship of the garment and ourselves. So many closets of my clients are overstuffed with items that are unworn because they don't flatter them. Anne had dozens of items that were beautiful, brand new, never worn designer garments that most would kill for, but they didn't flatter her coloring, shape, or features. In fact, they often accentuated shape imbalances by making her look more masculine, instead of feminine. For example, the shoulder pads and cut of the jacket made her look broader in the shoulders and narrower on the bottom, when the best shape would make her look curvier on the bottom and narrower on the top. Once you crack this code of 'style clarity', you will see your closet in a whole new light.

YOUR COLOR CLARITY

Meaning, what colors make your natural skin, hair, and eyes glow? Step one with my clients is draping them in various colors to determine which color palette best suits their skin. The 12-tonal system gives a personalized, accurate color palette. It's more precise than just autumn, winter, spring, and summer that you may have heard about from Color Me Beautiful. To accurately find out your color palette, the analysis must be done by a professional, but you can decide most of the other factors by yourself.

YOUR SHAPE CLARITY

Measuring my clients with a tape measure is step two in Define your shape clarity.

It's a painless process with me, I promise.

I factor in not just shoulder - to waist - to hip ratio but also your height and weight which makes the system very accurate. There are 48 different body types in this system, not 4-5 as most magazines would have you believe. Ignore the pear, apple, hourglass simplified 'types'. For example, you can't dress a tall, plus square the same as a petite, slim square. They are on totally different ends of the spectrum and the scale is different for each.

So once you know your exact shape prescription, I will be able to share with you exactly what cut of a dress, shirt, skirt, and pants will look best on you. It also tells you what kind of fabrics you should wear and which ones you should stay away from. And hemlines are also defined. This makes editing and shopping for your clothing so much easier. Necklines will be defined so you will know whether v neck, scoop neck, square neck, or off the shoulder will work best for your body. This information is applicable to all of your clothing and provides a road map for your style success. To accurately find out your shape prescription, the analysis has to be done by a professional, but you can decide most of the other factors by yourself.

YOUR ACCESSORIES

Your shape and color clarity will define what kinds of accessories will be best for you. For example, your eye color is a great accent color for accessories, and the undertone of your skin will dictate which metal - gold, rose gold, silver, or pewter - is the best for you. The scale of the accessory is dependent on your size. If you are on the small size, you don't want to wear oversized accessories, unless you want them to look like they are wearing you and not the other way around.

Iris Apfel is an example of the opposite of this principle. Her style is about exaggeration and making a massive statement so, as a small woman, she is wearing accessories that dwarf her.

I don't recommend this for non-celebrities.

The shape of your face is also a factor, and will give us information like - oval face shape does well with tear drop dangly earrings. A rectangular shaped face does well with small studs. Knowing your face shape is helpful information because when you are shopping, you will know what accessories will flatter your face. And as you are going through your accessories in your closet, it will explain why you don't wear certain accessories.

WHAT VISUAL MESSAGE ARE YOU SENDING?

Speaking of color...black pants can be another example similar to t-shirts. If they aren't special enough or cut beautifully, or paired with something exceptional, they can start to look a bit common and uniform-like. I know that many other style books have praised the value of black pants, but hey I just don't see it. For a couple reasons, really. Everyone knows this style cheat. It's so common to wear black pants and a shirt. It doesn't look unique. And also a large percent of the North American population has the same skin, hair, and eye coloring, and black is NOT a flattering color on them. And having a big contrast between the top garment with the lower half is often too overpowering for their natural coloring.

Once you know what colors work for you, it makes editing your closet a breeze and shopping so much easier. When you are scratching your head about why an item isn't doing it for you, ask yourself if the color flatters your face or brings it down. Most times, it's not the right color for you. And, sadly, black isn't everyone's style friend.

I so wish that this step was teachable, but this is best done with a color analysis professional such as myself. Give me a call to schedule your session. My contact info is in the back of this book.

YOUR PERSONAL STYLE

Does it represent your unique blend of style? Does it feel like you energetically? It could be a great outfit, but if it doesn't feel like you, it will never feel comfortable. When working with a private client, I often show them items that they would normally overlook. Most of the time, trying on something outside of their comfort zone is an AHA moment, but occasionally they aren't 'feeling it', and that is usually when 'energetically' the garment isn't speaking to my client. And so we move on.

Factoring in which styles fit your life and vibe is the third part of your style prescription.

There is no need to feel that you must be only one style. You can get creative here.

Ellen came to me loving so many different types of styles. She loved classic, bohemian, rock, hipster, cool, over the top. There really wasn't a style she didn't get excited about. I found her passion really inspiring because she had so much personality. But her coloring called for soft autumnal colors, and her shape was tall, full triangle which meant that, as a size 14-16, her hips were wider than her shoulders, so we needed to balance her figure out to appear like an hourglass.

And she loved all these fun styles that were trendy. But I knew if we went crazy out there with the garments, she might appear like a fashion victim and solicit ridicule in her competitive field. I made a suggestion that we stick to classic clothing styles and silhouettes, and let her accessories bring in all the flair and personality. So bold scarves, dramatic purses, edgy earrings, or bohemian jewelry. It was the right way to go and worked for her work travel schedule. She often found herself entertaining music celebrities for work, so we found some dramatic pieces that worked for her body and look.

Check out the Define your Style Intentions exercise in the workbook to learn about your own style musings. (Download your workbook at AlexandraStylist.com/workbook).

YOUR LIFESTYLE

Lifestyle is very important to factor into your style prescription because we take stock in where your life is right now. Once you define this, then it is factored into what needs to get edited out of your life, and what is missing and needs to be shopped for.

What are your daily needs, style wise?

What do you need to dress for?

How often are you at each home?

How much travel are you doing?

Is your life casual or dressy most of the time?

What percent of your life are you in an urban setting?

What percent of your life are you in a country setting?

What are your work/life style obligations?

How often do you need to wear black tie outfits?

Are you willing to repeat black tie outfits, or would you like to explore clothing rental?

My client Martha was living between her vineyard in Sonoma County and a country house in Pawling, New York. As a younger woman she ballroom danced for about 7 years so she had a whole closet full of gowns. Her current lifestyle was very casual - mostly California casual and then wintery casual. She spent most of her days in gardening clothing. If her and her husband went out socially, she wore slacks and a jacket or a casual dress. They didn't go to many parties anymore. It became clear to me, based on her current lifestyle, she had no need for her gowns. I found a wonderful place for her to donate them and have a second life. She felt much lighter after they left her house and made room for a proper coat closet.

You gravitate towards classics and basics but one day you realize that your uniform of jeans and a t-shirt, or yoga pants and a t-shirt, isn't doing you any favors. Let's say you go to run an errand in your uniform. You may not be excited to run into a friend or work colleague because you don't feel your best foot is forward. You see how great Diane Lane and other celebrities look in their Gap t-shirts and think that can work for you, too. But then you catch a glimpse of yourself in a window or a mirror and think, "Is that me?"

Getting real about where your life is at now is going to be useful information in defining how your closet should be stocked.

YOUR BUDGET

Knowing how much money you allocate to spend on new clothing every month, quarter, and year is a wonderful exercise to define where you should shop for new items. It's also good information to define where your cost per item threshold hits. You should also share this information with your personal stylist, so that you are on the same page. You can easily spend $10,000 or $10 on an item of clothing, depending on where you shop. Download the workbook now at AlexandrAStylist.com/workbook, and define your budget in the budget exercise.

It's very important to define for yourself the items that you are willing to spend more money on and that have more value to you. For example, in NYC, coats are very important to my clients because they're the first impression items. It's almost like your car, and has the power to elevate your style on a daily basis. Having a few signature statement coats is also a great way to communicate your style. But if you lived in a beach town, your most important items may be your bathing suit and caftans.

If your monthly budget is $1,000 for clothing, I would suggest staying away from places like Bergdorf Goodman, and focusing on Saks Fifth Avenue and consignment shops. Consignment shops are a wonderful way to supplement your closet with designer items at a fraction of the price. I would suggest giving them a thorough try on and inspection to make sure there isn't something wrong with the garment. Some designers have produced non-functional items in the past, like a summer weight, sleeveless top in a drab, depressing, winter-like color that makes you feel uninspired and confused on how to wear it. My client Anne had a muddy gray, silk, sleeveless top with tiny holes in it that we tried with all sorts of outfits before figuring out that it was seasonally challenged. It would never feel energetically right in the summer with white pants because of its muddy-like feeling to the color. But she would freeze if she wore it in the winter. It went in the donate/sell pile.

STYLE BY LOCATION

Lastly, define how you are going to manage your style in all your different locations.

Here are a few approaches to looking great in all of your homes.

Capsule Collection

You can choose to create a capsule collection of basics at every house based on weather, and then shuttle your accent accessories and jewelry between houses. Limit your color palette to 2 neutral colors and 2 accent colors. So, you can choose black and white as neutrals, and red and purple as accents. Or cream and tan as neutrals, and soft blue and pink as accents. Or black and navy as neutrals, and purple and red as accents.

With a capsule collection you can limit your items per category. For example, 5 pairs of pants.

3 pairs of jeans. 10 tops. 4 dresses. Keep all shoes and bags in a neutral or metallic palette.

You could also choose to pick one color per house. So at your Hamptons house, you only wear white with one accent color. And in NYC, you only wear black with an accent color. And in Paris, you only wear red. You could also make jeans the focus of your weekend home. This minimalist approach can save you a lot of headaches. This works well for a woman who is classic in style and prefers a more neutral palette.

ARE YOU A UNIFORM DRESSER OR A CHAMELEON?

Uniform

You can choose to create a simplified uniform for yourself. I have a client who only wears easy dresses in the summer months, and then in the winter she wears jeggings with tunics over it. She might also wear jeans from time to time, but it keeps things very simplified without having to stock lots of different kinds of garments. For example, do you really need shorts, culottes, skirts, or skorts? How can you have less and make it easier for you?

Melinda Gates's assistant contacted me a few years ago as they were looking for a full-time personal stylist for her life. I got a glimpse into her style preferences. Melinda keeps to a very simple uniform of basics, and with her favorite items she simply buys multiples and makes sure they are stocked at each house. So she has her favorite sunglasses at each house. When she travels she often has to adapt to the environment, so she needs more casual outfits with shorts when she is in Africa, but they need to be quality because she is meeting diplomats and dignitaries.

Chameleon

You can also choose to dress drastically differently at each house based on the vibe of the location. My Grandma Pat shared with me recently that her philosophy of going between 4 houses was as so: "If I was boring, I would dress the same at every house but I'm not, so I cater my clothing based on where I am. When I'm in Vermont I'm wearing pressed slacks, when I'm in Florida I'm dressier and more preppy, and when I'm in Maine I'm more nautical but I'm always dramatic."

So your Paris home could be stocked with more fashion forward, dramatic frocks, and your Hamptons house could be your refuge where you curl up in cozy knits, and your New York home could have your chic precise looks.

Your body, your style, your closets are a living breathing ever changing being. So how you stock your homes is up to you, and I'm here to help you create a roadmap and implement your big picture. Your closets should support your life wherever it is.

You have just finished the first step in the style prescription process: DEFINE. Once you have defined your style in all of its facets, it will give you criteria to base your detoxing and shopping decisions on. It's a strong filter to run your decisions through. Next up, I'm going to share my style philosophies with you, and then we will move onto the DETOX step.

CHAPTER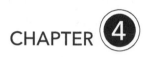

STYLE PHILOSOPHIES TO LIVE BY

Remember my client Anne? After working together one season, she saw dramatic changes in her life and style. We sent her jeans and t-shirts to 'summer camp', i.e. another closet in her NYC house, to have a break. She started wearing the beautiful things in her closet. We cleared away anything she wasn't wearing which was A LOT. She was no longer reaching for black items of clothing, and her husband complimented her on her soft colors. He could see her femininity more clearly. We sent a rack of full outfits to her Palm Beach house and she shared with me things she had worn or not. Based on our editing her NYC closet, she edited her Palm Beach closet with ease and instantly felt lighter.

After two seasons of working together, she reported that she was liking having less choices in her closet. For the first time in her life, she and her husband had a two week planned vacation in Europe. We packed her for the trip and made outfits for every occasion. It was the first time she was relaxed before a trip and was delighted to be organized and prepared. She wore most everything on the trip, and it was a huge success. When she shopped by herself, she was making better choices for herself and choosing items that were flattering to her face and body.

She was also able to create outfits for herself with ease, and started to experiment more.

Her closet was no longer stressful to her. During our months of working together, Anne was able to digest crucial style philosophies and have tremendous success with her closet. Style philosophies help when you are trying to figure out what to wear. In this chapter, I'm going to share with you the most powerful style philosophies so that you can apply them to your closet.

STYLE PHILOSOPHIES TO PONDER:

Confidence is Key

You can be wearing the most beautiful outfit in the world, but if it's doesn't feel like you, you won't exude confidence. And that's a shame because others may pick up on this nuance. So, it's important to wear things that energetically feel like you, and then you can wear them with confidence.

Be Comfortable in Your Style No Matter Where You Are in the World

One of the things I hear over and over is, "I want to be comfortable." No one in all 16 years of my styling career has wanted to suffer for fashion. Which is funny to me…but also telling that the fashion industry is missing the mark on most women. We ALL want to be comfortable, to move, stretch, and possibly feel as if we could dance in our outfits. That's probably why Juicy Couture sweat suits were as successful as they were. And Lululemon is a runaway success. And why a common complaint in Marin County, California from women is that they don't know how to get out of their yoga pants; they are THAT comfortable.

It's important to be comfortable but not so much that it makes you feel schleppy. That's the philosophy.

No One Remembers Normal

When I started working with Laura, who works in tech sales and travels frequently for work, she confided in me that she was passed over for a promotion recently. When we first took a look at her closet, which was filled with black and white and hardly any color, I asked her if she was shy or an introvert. She said no, just the opposite. I scratched my head. Do you like color, I asked her? Absolutely, she said. I love color and print, I just have never known what to buy. I could see how there was a huge disconnect between who she was, and the closet that was in front of me. When we went shopping, all the fun prints and colors were what she was gravitating towards. So we built her a wardrobe with fun, but work-appropriate outfits. She hadn't realized that she was dressing without color. But now with all the outfits having tons of personality, she started to really shine. And here's what she said a year after working together,

"It's been over a year since I had a style makeover with Alexandra, and the benefits keep accruing! Never have I felt so confident and comfortable in my style. And, with the tools and knowledge she gave me, I have been able to buy more flattering clothes to supplement the ones she and I selected, which I am mostly still wearing, even though I lost 15 pounds! Does she know how to plan ahead, or what?! Working with Alexandra was truly a life-changing experience. With her combination of style savvy, fit expertise, and deep understanding of your personality and budget, she will empower you to show your best self to the world. I wish all women could feel as good as I do every day, when I look in my closet and wonder, what perfect outfit should I wear today?"

The point of this story is to let you know that it's much more powerful to dress and feel like yourself. Dressing for yourself and your own joy is the highest form of personal style. There is no need to blend in or dress 'normal', unless that is your personality.

Dress for the Life You Want, Not for the One You Have

Joanne came to me while she was working as the head of PR for a major bank here in NYC. She had held that position for a while and was ready for her next big job. Her weekends were spent on Nantucket with her family. We started working together, and as we were in the shopping part of the process, she told me about a huge opportunity that she was interviewing for as head of PR for a major beauty conglomerate. Luckily, we were already focusing on her style becoming more feminine and fashion forward, and less corporate. When it came time for her interview with the chairman of the company, she had this fantastic skirt suit to wear with the perfect shoes, bag, and jewelry. She simply looked the part of head of PR for a beauty company. She nailed the interview, got the job, and is still happy in her post and her new wardrobe.

I have seen this happen with countless clients where we start working together, and then they start to attract new opportunities that really excite them. As you ponder your style, you can focus more on where you want to be in life, not where you are at. You want your business to be 'in the black', dress the part of a successful business owner. You want to speak at events, dress the way a speaker would dress. You want to lead, dress as a leader. Dressing the part allows you to feel the confidence and the power of possibility.

"Fashion fades. Style is eternal" YSL

During the detox process of working with Anne, we edited out dozens of pieces that could be put into the very trendy category. They were items that had crazy embellishments and odd proportions, and weren't flattering to her figure. Through the process, we discovered that her innate style was more classic and simple.

When you are looking at your wardrobe, do you see a reflection of yourself in the clothing and accessories?

Or do they feel like strangers to you?

If you don't have a wardrobe that is in alignment with your true nature, it won't feel right when you get dressed.

Most women don't do well with trendy clothing.

You may even feel like an imposter.

Your face won't be happy, and then you won't know what to wear or how to fix the issue.

And we don't want that to happen.

Party Where You Are at Style Wise

"Party where you are." I adapted this phrase from Marie Forleo. To me, it means taking stock of exactly where you are, accepting it, moving on, and letting the world know that you're not going to let anything about it stop you.

Sarah came to me halfway through her weight loss journey. She had lost about 75 pounds and was on track to lose some more, but she realized she didn't want to wait to get her style to the next level. She was sick of frumpy, tent-like clothing and wanted to dazzle. She signed up for my style makeover program, and we got to work. It was inspiring to see her shine in her new style. She reported that she started to get compliments from her friends - something that was new to her. Accepting herself, and working with a stylist was the best decision, because she could look her best now, not months from now. There is power in meeting yourself exactly where you are right NOW.

The Only Thing Constant is Change

Another fabulous client, Lisa, came to me after having lost 100 pounds and recovering from cancer. She lives in Upstate New York but was currently staying with her parents during and post radiation. She had a condensed version of her closet in the city. She was still losing weight going through chemo, but she had decided now was the time to work with me. When she called me, my practice was full with a waiting list for a few months, so I referred her to a colleague of mine but a few months later, she called me again and was insistent on working with me. Luckily, I had a slot open so we started working together. She knew things were going to change with her body, but she didn't care. She wanted to be prepared and to look good for all that life would throw at her. We soon joked that some outfits were for 'from chemo to cafe' instead of the usual 'from day to night'. We focused on affordable brands because we knew her size would keep changing. She went from a size 22 to 18, to 16 to a 14, and she is still losing weight. She ended up spending more time in New York, so she edited her upstate closet and moved most of her stuff to the city where we sorted through it together. She loves that she has outfits already created that she knows will make her feel good when she needs a boost. She shared with me that she thinks every woman deserves to feel this good. Life will always hand us changes and evolutions, so why not get support during every stage of the process?

Acceptance

The most important concept is Acceptance – accepting where your body, life, and coloring is today. How many of you struggle with getting rid of things from your closet because they were expensive, even when they no longer support you or your life? For example, if you no longer attend black tie dinners, why not donate your gowns to a school theatre program where they can be used and given a second life?

I've watched a Californian client struggle with this issue. We were editing her closet when we came upon these Manolo Blahnik ankle tie black heels. I give her credit. She was a trendsetter for Manolos – before Sex and the City! She immediately got super attached and said we couldn't get rid of the heels. But, she had maybe worn them twice since purchasing them 20 years ago. Plus, she spends most of her time these days gardening, going to the gym, or taking her puppy to the playground. Here's what I suggested since they held so much meaning for her: Display the shoes out of the box on the shelf as ART and appreciate them every day.

My clients have shared with me that dressing for errands, the farmers' market, the gym, and other downtimes is the hardest challenge. Let's say you find yourself walking the dog a lot. Why not build flattering outfits appropriate for that activity?

Most women would love to be the desired hourglass shape. Only 8% of women are this shape. My job is to create the illusion of this shape, which I teach my clients how to do.

How many of you have clothing in your closet that:

Isn't the right size or color?

No longer serves your current lifestyle?

Is older than 10 years?

Has never been worn?

We all can relate. But we can also all take steps toward acceptance, and with it, change.

There comes a time in your style journey when acceptance is important. Accepting of your body and where you are. Accepting of your age. Not being able to accept that your body has changed is one of the number one style blocks I have seen women experience. They don't fit into an item anymore but they don't want to get rid of it, because they think they are going to fit into it again. Here's the thing. I want you to have a closet filled with items that work and support your life NOW, as it is. In future chapters, I'm going to share with you some strategies for phasing items out of your life that are less painful than just tossing them.

Define Who You Are Dressing For
(Download your workbook at AlexandrAStylist.com/ workbook and complete this exercise now)

Figuring out who you are getting dressed for every day is important.

Are you dressing for yourself?

To feel good?

To feel sexy, or to feel comfortable?

Are you dressing to impress people at work or your clients?

Are you dressing for your husband, to please him?

What do you immediately need?

Are you missing a top to a specific skirt or pant?

What kind of event stressed you out because you had nothing to wear?

What kinds of outfits do you need stocked here?

How often are you at this house?

How many outfits do you need realistically?

If you only spend weekends here and have washing help, do you need a large quantity of outfits?

Are you dressing for the overall style or theme at this house?

If you can't think of some styles, I've provided some ideas for you here: beachy casual, or urban chic, eco casual, country casual, woodsy comfortable, relaxed, bright colors and prints, beach chic.

What colors would work best to wear?

What's missing clothing wise?

Any special activity wear?

What accessories do you need stocked here? Purses, jewelry, shrugs, scarves, coats, gloves?

Do this exercise for every house or trip you have planned in the next year. It will help you forecast your needs and get you prepared, so that you can get dressed for any occasion that may pop up.

Wonderful! Armed with these new philosophies I'm sure you will start seeing your closet and world around you with different eyes. You might notice other women on the street and how they are dressed. Or you may begin to see why you haven't been wearing certain items in your closets, even if they were expensive gifts. Now let's tackle the second step in the style prescription process: DETOX.

CHAPTER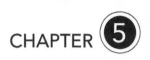

DETOX

efore you shop for one item make sure you clean out all your closets and get closet clarity. This is no easy feat when you have multiple closets and homes.

"When in doubt throw it out."

Americans are acquiring more and more stuff, and the average American house is bursting at the seams. It's easy to consume and buy, and not so easy to shed and lighten your load. Especially when you have multiple homes and closets. It's easy to have the attitude 'out of sight, out of mind', and often you may not spend very much time at a certain house. I have a client who only spends occasional weekends at their Hamptons home, so her time is so limited when she is there.

The art and practice of detoxing and getting rid of items can be very therapeutic if you see it that way. As we are going through their closets, many clients will rediscover forgotten items and find money or items of worth to sell. They are also energetically making space in their life for new things, people, and opportunities to come in. They often discover lost items at one of their houses that had been long forgotten. I use clearing out to go to the next level in my business. The less clutter I have, the more productive I am.

My client Sarah splits her time between her Upstate New York country home and a pied-à-terre in the city. When we started together, she was not working and hadn't shopped for clothing in years. She had a lot of dated pieces of her wardrobe and was wearing a fraction of her clothing. I found out that she was keeping old, tired items at her country home that weren't getting much wear. She did some closet clearing up there too. Right after we cleared Sarah's closet of bags full of old clothing, mostly suits she wasn't wearing, she got the job opportunity of a lifetime heading up a department at a major art museum. She had not been working for a couple years. Is this a coincidence? I think not! The work is powerful if you do the work.

With multiple houses and multiple closets, I suggest detoxing them one at a time, or one season at a time. You're going to want to chunk the project down to digestible bits at your own pace. If you prefer to work in big bursts, do that. If you're better as a plodder, do bits at a time. Do your main residence first, and then attack the next home which needs the most help second.

I also recommend to my clients that each house have a designated LOVING NOW closet that is stocked with everything you are loving and wearing now. Then your other closets can have coats, out of season, and black tie outfits.

The point is to narrow what you look at every day and to have those key items all in one spot for easy access. You might choose to travel or shuttle these LOVING NOW items between homes or purchase duplicates.

Detoxing your closets BEFORE you shop is also key because it allows you to make space in your closet and to take stock of what you have and what items might need a mate. You know, that skirt that never gets worn because you don't have a top that goes with it. Especially if that skirt is at a weekend home that doesn't get much use.

Tip: As you are editing your closets, keep a notebook or your cell phone handy to jot down notes for your wardrobe master plan. You want to note items that you realize are missing pieces or would complete outfits in your closets. You might want to make a note for each house.

For example - espresso, long sleeve top to go with printed pants. Earrings to go with Fendi dress.

This list of items is going to be your STYLE SHOPPING LIST, which will help you when you are shopping for new pieces so that you stay on track and avoid your past style blind spots. Copy your style shopping lists in your cell phone notes so that it will be with you everywhere.

Shopping becomes an easy, grazing-like activity, and you can check online or pop in shops as it works for your schedule. And if you are curious to see my client's transformations, I've included some links inside the workbook about that, as well.

If you haven't downloaded the workbook yet, make sure you do so now, as there will be more exercises throughout the book to complement your experience. Now would be a great time to complete the Define your Wardrobe Master plan for each of your homes by downloading the workbook at AlexandrAStylist.com/workbook.

My process to detox your closet with ease is as follows:

1. Define: Clarify what looks good on you (which you have already done in the previous chapter.) A personal stylist who is trained in color and shape analysis can help with this step immensely, as we often cannot objectively view ourselves.

2. Prep: Gather garbage bags and racks to make your detox process easier. Label bags toss, donate, give away, and that way, you will have a place for every piece as you decide to send it to its new life. Yes, what you are doing in this step is giving your items which were idle and lonely a chance for a new life with a new owner who will hopefully cherish and use the items and wear them out.

3. Vision Boards: If you're into arts and crafts, a physical vision board is fun to make. You may choose to make a vision board for each house if you define yourself as a chameleon. Pinterest board is a digital version and just as great, and you can link to actual pieces that you may buy. I have a video about how to create a vision board using Pinterest for you, go to AlexandrAStylist.com/pinterest-opt-in. The vision board will give a reference of your style and look. It's useful while detoxing and shopping. For example,

if your desired style on your vision board is mainly filled with classic items and you come across a heavy metal rocker jacket that hasn't been worn in years, you know it's not meant for you anymore. It's time for it to find a new home where it will be worn and cherished. The memories may stop you emotionally, but you can also snap a picture of it and put it on social media to keep it in your heart and mind.

4. Detox: Start by taking every item in your closet out onto a rack or your bed to sort. You want to make sure to touch and go through every item. This takes time and you may have to do it in big chunks of items, but it's worth it. As you are going through, you are asking yourself:

    ~   Have I been wearing this?
    ~   Is it a good color and shape for me?
    ~   Should this live at another home of mine?

Some common style blocks that I see get in the way of a client's progress in this step are the following:

The Blind Spot

We all have our style blind spots. Meaning the items we purchase multiple of and never realize that we don't really wear the items. They are also the items you bring home from the department store, not realizing you have multiples at home already. It's comfortable to just buy that black top. For some, it's a white top. Feels safe and secure. But then at home, you go "well that was silly, I have a bunch at home." But it's a basic so you keep it. I find these 'style blind spot' items accumulate over time, and they take up a lot of space. That's one of the parts of the closet I help my clients weed through. With Anne, it was black pants. She had over 20 pairs of black pants and none of them she was really wearing. It's hard to edit out this blind spot because they are generally basic items you believe will be of use and that you will need them. But that is fear-based because we now have washing machines, and unless you wear a uniform, it's really not helping you. You're going to want to pay special attention when you are detoxing your closet, as you will most likely find a dozen of basically the same type of item that doesn't get a ton of wear. You will identify the blind spot, detox the items, and move on wiser in the process.

Favorites - Friend or Frenemy?

Anne originally called me because she found herself wearing the same jeans and t-shirt every day despite having beautifully organized multiple closets full of designer clothing. Unlike most of my clients, she had so many closets that you could see everything she had; clothes were not bursting out. There was space between every garment, but they were still not getting worn. In her case, her favorite items were getting lots of wear, but all of her dressier items were mostly unworn.

She was paralyzed by the sheer number of options.

For her case, more was NOT better.

So she would return over and over to her jeans and t-shirts.

What message is a t-shirt sending?

Does it say, "I'm successful?" In LA, it's almost cool to dress down if you are successful.

But in NYC, the t-shirt isn't putting your best foot forward.

The problem with favorites, after we have worn them to death, is that we are emotionally attached to the items and have stopped seeing them objectively.

We don't see the pills.

We don't realize they're tired.

We don't realize they need to be retired.

I wondered if Anne's upbringing was casual. Or if she didn't feel at home in the Upper East Side. I knew that she had been a downtown girl when she was single, and she was now living uptown. Which in Manhattan are entirely different worlds. So no wonder she was feeling out of sorts. Her unconscious block had her more comfortable dressed down, and it was hard for her to reach for the really nice items in her closet. She shared with me once that she went to reach for a really high-end piece and she heard a voice in her head that said, "Don't touch that." As if it was too nice for her. We might not even be aware that our early programming is affecting our style. The voices may never leave, but we can choose to turn the volume down and say to the voice, "I hear you, but I'm going for a new choice." Her new awareness enabled her to break her style habits and start dressing in a new way.

Emotional Style Blocks

During the DETOX process, we will most likely stumble upon items with sentimental value. Those that are no longer worn now because they don't fit or aren't age appropriate but the memories are so strong, it's hard to let go of them. Here are some of the phrases I've heard:

"That was a gift from my _____. I can't possibly give it away"

"I wore that when I met my husband. I can't possibly get rid of it"

"I was 20 when I used to wear that. I can wear that when I lose 5 pounds"

I encourage my clients to embrace the now - "party where they are at" and let go of anything not supporting their life now. If you are pregnant, it's a totally different scenario. You might want to check out Le Tote in the resources section that allows you to shop, wear, and return maternity wear. Which is perfect for pregnant women.

I made a whole video about emotional roadblocks with clearing out your closet inside my Closet Clarity program. You can watch at AlexandrAStylist.com/emotional-rescue.

Donate/Give/Sell/Toss - Getting Items Out of Your Homes

Giving away items to friends or family members can make the detoxing feel easier, because you are improving their lives. Make sure to only gift items that you know they want and will wear. After you take items out of your closet, the sheer number of items may shock you, and it might be hard to immediately get them out the door. You can move them to a rack in another room for a week of resting. And then see if you miss any items. Revisit the items after a week or two to see if you made the right choice. Most times you have, but occasionally there might be a piece that is needed for a particular outfit.

Once you have decided to pay the items forward, make sure to actually get the bags out of your homes before you dip back into them. I have had clients keep the items on a rack for a transitional period to see if they might need an item here or there. This is only applicable to items that are in wonderful condition. Ratty and tired items should be discarded immediately.

See the resources section in the back of the book for where to donate, sell, or gift your detoxed items.

So you've detoxed your closet, but how do you keep it looking this way? The next step to detoxing is learning how to maintain.

MAINTENANCE

Have you ever returned to a home after a long time, like a year, and opened the closets but nothing feels like you? This would happen when I would leave things at one of my parents' homes with years of hiatus. The silver lining was I was no longer emotionally attached to the items, so it was now so easy to detox them.

Maintaining closets and homes are something you help along daily, weekly and monthly.

I recommend to my clients that when they purchase some new items they consider matching the amount to go out of their closet. A one for one system. This way the closet stays even keeled.

Organize

"If you can't see it, you won't wear it." ASG

Now that you have more space in your closet because you have purged some items…right…you've given some stuff away… I want you to think strategically about how your closet can be organized in a way that supports your current lifestyle.

Yeah, you get a fresh start here!

There are many ways to organize your closets, and you get to decide what works for you.

The most important concept of organization is to tailor it to you, your needs, lifestyle, and different homes. Design your closet organization based on your daily and weekly life. If you wear ball gowns regularly, make sure they are easy to access. If you are in a bathing suit and caftan daily, make sure those are prominent. Make sense?

The most popular way with my clients is to organize by GARMENT type and then by color.

For example, all of your dresses hang together, all your pants hang together, and then within each category you organize from light to dark color wise.

Picking a system will help.

Every client, closet, and home are unique.

Try to pick one system and use it in all of your homes for continuity and habit.

If you only keep a few outfits at a certain house, you might just want to organize most simply by COLOR.

Here are 3 other different concepts to reorganize:

The LOVING NOW section is a dedicated area with everything you are jamming on and wearing now. All items should be in season. You want to be able to access your underwear, socks, jewelry and accessories so that you can properly get dressed quickly. And it should be placed in the part of your closet that is easiest to access. This will be your main closet where you are stocked to fully get dressed and organized.

If you are currently in between seasons, or live in a place where the temperature fluctuates dramatically during the day - for example Palm Springs, you want to have a mix of warm weather and cold weather in the same closet. Make sure you have your favorites there so that you can make quick decisions. Sometimes it's better to have less in the LOVING NOW closet because it won't cause style overwhelm.

Your extra closets can be relegated to coat closet, out of season closets, formal wear and black tie attire. I have a client who is a performer and so her most prominent easy to access LOVING NOW section is the gowns that she performs in, and all the other casual wear takes second priority. Her closet is organized differently than say one of my executive clients who has to impress in the corporate world. Her LOVING NOW section is work dresses with jackets.

If you know mornings are stressful, you might want to plan 4 outfits in advance on Sunday night and hang them in your LOVING NOW department. So think about your daily style and environment needs or by rainbow of COLOR, so all your black things together, all cream things together.

My clients who love color do it this way because then dressing monochromatically becomes easy. Or you organize by SEASON. I have a client blessed with three closets, so we put all of her LOVING NOW in her main walk-in closet and put off season and formal clothing in the bedroom closet because it suits her current needs. You can tailor your homes and your closets to your needs. And once you've chunked it out by section, you can sub organize by color or garment type.

If you filled out your inventory part of the worksheets, you will be able to gauge what organizational tools you will need and how much to buy since you will have detailed info.

What might you need?

~   Built in custom closet?
~   Shoe organizers?
~   Some accessory displays?
~   Clear jewelry boxes?
~   Some hooks?

It's best to be able to see everything you have - that way you will wear them.

Get those shoes and jewelry out of the boxes they came in.

Swap out shoe boxes for clear display boxes.

Check out the resources chapter for my favorite services and tools.

A few key products and hacks that make organizing your closets a breeze:

~ Hanging hooks behind a leaning mirror on the wall will hide your handbag storage.

~ You can also hang your bags using hanging space with shower curtain hooks.

~ Ideally you want all of your in season shoes in one area on a rack or built in shelves.

~ Shoe trees will help prolong the life of your shoes especially the delicate leather ones.

~ Boot trees are necessary, as your boots are the first to start showing wear from sitting folded upon itself.

~ Do not store shoes in the boxes they came in because you won't be able to see them quickly.

~ Store out of season shoes in clear boxes from the Container Store. I prefer this solution to Polaroid pictures on the outside of shoe boxes.

~ Some type of scarf storage is helpful so that you can see every option. I prefer rolling them and then stacking them in a box on its side, but a close second is a scarf organizer by Umbra from the container store.

~ Use one big ring to store all of your camisoles in the closet.

A few key tips:

~ A bulletin board makes a wonderful way to display your costume jewelry so that you actually wear it.

~ Store your valuable jewelry in a locked box.

~ Use side walls to install little rods and store your sunglasses there.

~ Knits (sweaters and tops) should be folded so they retain their shape. If knits are hung, they will stretch out and won't last as long.

~ Don't have time to run to the Container Store for scarf boxes? Turn an open shoebox horizontally and on the side and use it to roll up scarves inside that way you can see your options.

~ Create a check in / check out station at each home. A dedicated area where you can see the smaller items you need to access to get out the door. Keys, scarves, gloves, hats, jewelry, wallet, purses, lipgloss, Kleenex, etc. should all be nicely organized and visible for you to grab and go. If you always store your keys in the same place, they won't get lost.

~ Aim to have an inch between hangers. This is a nice goal that not everyone is able to achieve but is nice to strive towards.

~ Once a week create a week of outfits for you to wear and hang them on a standing rod. This works for those who like to plan.

~ To make organizing your closets at multiple houses easier to navigate, choose one type of organization and stick to it at each house.

~ Send certain items to each house based on use, and let them live there.

For example, Anne has all of her casual, cozy, neutral color beach wear in her Hamptons house, because they are very low key and don't entertain out there. It is organized by COLOR. She has most of her dressy and colorful outfits in Palm Beach, because they are very social down there. So her Palm Beach home is sorted by COLOR and outfits hang together for simplicity. Her 5th avenue house has her urban and chic type outfits. She has one big walk in closet organized by GARMENT type and then sorted by color. It is stocked with all of her undergarments, workout wear, bags, jewelry and accessories for New York. Her check in / check out station lives there. She only turns her closet over twice a year instead of four. She realized in working with me that trying to define things in four seasons was too complicated, so now she thinks of her closet as Fall/Winter which is mild/cold and Spring/Summer which is warm/hot. The closet in another bedroom is stocked with out of season clothing and black tie outfits. A hall closet has her coats and winter accessories. Each house is stocked with a different defined style. She is able to be a chameleon based on where she is in the world.

Detoxing before shopping is crucial because it makes you aware of what you have and what you don't have. Knowing this, you can go out and start shopping, because you'll no longer be buying clothes you don't need and that don't fit your style. This may feel different to you because in the past when you thought about your style you started with shopping. My process is set up so that you start with a clean slate and on the right foot to shop with success.

CHAPTER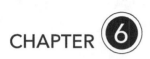

SHOP FOUNDATIONS

When I say foundations I mean the most important foundation of your outfit…your undergarments.

And specifically your bras, underwear, hosiery, and shapewear.

They can easily be the most important part of your outfit.

The wrong bra can make you look dumpy and the wrong underwear can make you look sloppy.

The right shape wear can instantly make you look slimmer and the wrong one can add weight.

Your twins need the right support so they can look amazing in that top or dress.

The first item to start shopping for? Your undergarments.

How often do you throw out and purchase new bras?

You may realize that you have bras sitting unworn at each home.

Do you travel with your favorite bras and lingerie?

You are going to think I'm crazy when I tell you that the average lifespan of a bra is 6-9 months.

Not years!

But it also depends on a bunch of factors like quality of the bra, if it's been rotated, and what kind of care it has received.

That means that most women are walking around in DEAD bras, and in your case, these bras may be sitting in your homes unworn.

Here are some indications that your bra is dead and should be tossed:

~ The elastic is stretched out
~ You're wearing it on the last hook and it's still moving around and loose
~ Your body has changed and you are wearing the wrong size
~ The wires are poking out
~ Your boobs are hanging lower than they should
~ There are holes in the bra
~ The hook is broken

If you use all of your homes equally, I would suggest having 3-5 everyday bras at each house that you rotate wearing because wearing the same bra every day will drastically reduce its lifespan. If you have a house that you only use once a year do not store bras there.

You might want to include your sexier pieces at your beach house or specific foundational pieces for certain outfits. For example, strapless bras are much needed in tropical climates.

You also might just want to travel with your favorite bras and not choose to stock your homes with bras. That way you can keep an eye on the ones you have and replace them as needed.

With multiple homes you actually have an opportunity to express yourself with lingerie depending on the locale. If you are comfortable being a chameleon, you might find yourself wearing a brighter or sexier color in the tropics, but in New York or your city home, sticking to nude and black colors. Feel free to define each house as a different lingerie identity. Channel Bridget Bardot in St. Barts and Dita Von Tease in Paris. Have fun with it!

You also might decide to stock a particular home with more sexy lingerie because you know you will have more opportunities for intimate moments. Sometimes the pace of the city gets to us, but when we're in a tropical setting we can let loose and feel free. Also in warmer climates you're going to want to have at least two strapless bras for those more bare dresses. And possibly specific Spanx for white pants or more form fitting dresses.

Never put your bras in the washing machine. Hand wash them with delicate wash by the Laundress or another bra friendly detergent. Line dry. If you do put them in the washer make sure to put them in a mesh bag, use delicate cycle, and then line dry.

When should you get refit for a new bra?

~ You haven't worn the bra for over a year since it's been hiding at a house
~ When your weight changes more than 10 pounds in either direction
~ Pregnancy
~ Menopause
~ Illness
~ Hormonal shifts
~ You haven't been at that home in over a year.

To be safe it's good to get refit every 6-12 months. Before you start shopping, you're going to want to consult your style shopping list to see what you need for each home.

Remember, we talked about your style shopping list in Chapter 5.

The right bra can give you an instant lift and make all of your clothing more flattering. This is always the first stop shopping wise in my process, because if the bra isn't fitting right - the outfit won't look right.

The following are some tips when it comes to undergarments.

To Spanx or Not

I have some clients who love how Spanx look on them. Most women don't like the feeling of being squeezed like a sausage, but it's worth it to some and not to others. Wearing Spanx is a personal decision.

A few years ago my boyfriend surprised me by sharing with me that his favorite part of my body was what I would call my pooch. He loved it because it was soft. I was shocked! Here was this body part that for years I felt could be flatter and wished it was flatter, and it was perfect to him.

It changed my whole perspective on the need for Spanx and I decided to start loving that body part, instead of wishing it would stomach crunch away.

If Spanx makes you feel better and you like the look there are so many wonderful options to choose from. My favorite bra and foundation resources in NYC are included in my second book Vetted by a Stylist. You can check it out here VettedbyaStylist.com

They can help you find the perfect undergarments for those items that need it. Spanx isn't the only company.

Hosiery

Hose are also very personal items.

What to wear for hose if you have open toe shoes?

I, for example, prefer to wear hose even in Miami, but I have discovered toe-less hose that I wear with open toe shoes. It gives the support and sweat management of hose but without toes, so they look normal in my wedge sandals. You might want to stock your warm weather residences with toe-less hose. Spanx can really help under summer weight white pants.

True fact: Spanx were born because founder Sara Blakely cut the feet off a pair of panty hose to wear underneath a pair of white summer pants.

In the colder areas like Aspen you're going to want to have extra long underwear, cashmere tights, and sweater dresses handy so that you can look good and feel warm. The other hose that my clients and I love is the micro mesh stocking by Hue. It's like a fishnet and a hose had a baby. They are subtly sexy and I have gotten countless compliments from men.

How Can I Be Sexy but Not Slutty?

Wearing garter belts and stay up thigh high stockings are sexy but sometimes wearing them isn't as comfortable as the micro mesh.

Most of My Wardrobe is Black; How Can I Infuse Some Color?

Fun colored tights are a great way to add a pop of color but for some it may feel too Punky Brewster. I recommend it for those under 40, and for the rest of us stick to neutrals like nude, brown, and black. Yes, brown is a wonderful neutral tight if black is too harsh. White tights often look nurse like.

Now that you've got your foundation of foundations solidly laid, you can move onto the fun part -shopping! Hopefully if you don't like to shop, I can make it a bit easier and stress free for you in the next chapter.

CHAPTER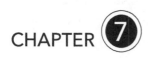

SHOP

n this chapter I'm going to teach you why shopping is broken, how to maximize your shopping experience, shop like a pro, decide whether to shop high-end designer, mass market or bespoke.

WHY SHOPPING IS BROKEN

Shopping!

Some women love to shop.

And some women hate to shop.

Generally, as a stylist I hear from the women who hate to shop because they need help with it.

And it seems the more closets and more homes a woman has, the more challenging it can be to know what to shop for.

You look at all that you have and wonder why you can't make an outfit that feels like you.

I get it!

Stores are big, confusing, and hard to navigate.

Staff may tell you things that mess with your mind. You buy that outfit they say looks amazing on you, and then you get it home and it doesn't feel right. You're not sure what sizes to pick or what designers to look at. Or what shops to go into. You go in to get an outfit for tomorrow's party, but you get sidetracked and end up with nothing remotely that will work. And online is more confusing than ever. Your head is swimming because you have events in different locations, and you're not sure what you have in each place. Or if you have complete outfits with the right accessories there.

Why Personal Shoppers Can Suck
(not all are terrible)

Personal shoppers at department stores are trained to sell merchandise.

And lots of it.

They make money based on how much you spend.

Personal shoppers also have no idea what is already in your closet.

The only information they go on is what you tell them and it's often difficult for them to grasp your style quickly. Personal shoppers are not trained to teach you what looks good on you. They often haven't gotten the scientific training to educate you in that manner.

Yes, the information is based on science - color science and shape analysis. Such un-sexy terms, I know!! I've been in the dressing rooms with personal shoppers and a client when she has said, "You can never have too many pairs of black pants." When during our closet detox session, we have taken out multiple pairs of black pants because they send such a plain boring message.

There is more information about the difference between a personal stylist and a personal shopper on my blog at AlexandrAStylist.com/define-stylists-what-do-they-really-do/.

The Main Reason You Hate to Shop and How to Fix It

This week I was talking with a new potential client who shared with me how much she hates shopping. She described to me how she recently got a jacket for a speaking engagement. She went shopping with a friend and they saw one jacket that she liked, but it wasn't in her size. She didn't want to ask for it in her size. So her friend fought with her and then finally asked for it in her size. The jacket worked out but it made me realize something. So I asked her, "When you shop, how many items do you select to try on?" "One to three" was her response. Bingo! This is one of the main reasons why people hate shopping. They don't set themselves up for success in the dressing room. Some women solve this problem by hiring a personal stylist. Style, like dating, is a numbers game. When I pull for a client, I pull 1-2 racks of clothing. I stack the odds in my favor. If something doesn't work out there's no disappointment, because you didn't put all your style eggs in one basket.

Yesterday, I did a mini shop to get a few spring dresses with a lady who is very busty and knows pretty well what suits her. Together we found about 15 dresses to try on, and

3 were total winners. The whole process was quick because we both know her style really well, and I'm pretty good at this. We also figured out another key factor to dress shopping for her: she looks best in dresses that don't have a seam at the waist area. Because every time you shop it's another opportunity to see what works and why. So, next time you find yourself on a mission, get laser focused but pick out way more pieces than you need, so that you can narrow it down and take the pressure of that one dress working out.

How to Find What You Are Looking For

In this chapter, I'm going to take you through my process for shopping for my clients so that you can learn some strategies to make it successful.

How to Shop - Department Store vs. Designer Boutique

Start with the big department stores and if you like a designer who is stocked there see if they are carried at other big department stores by doing a quick search in their search box. And then visit those stores to see what they have from that designer. Often big department stores get exclusives on particular items or colors that another store may not have. And their own store has different merchandise, too.

HOW TO SHOP TO MAXIMIZE YOUR SUCCESS

Set Yourself Up for Success

1. ALLOW ENOUGH TIME There is nothing worse than shopping frantically with a deadline. You've got the pressure of finding the perfect thing for that event that everyone is going to be talking about. So instead of shopping just before you need something I love to get my clients set up for success by stocking their closets with everything they may need. But if you do have a deadline give yourself enough time to find it. Don't self sabotage your style success.

2. SCHEDULE IT AT THE BEST TIME OF DAY Schedule your shopping at a time during the day when you will be in an optimum state of mind. After a healthy meal is a good time. If you can bring a trusted objective friend or trusted stylist that is even better. I would suggest time blocks of 1-2.5 hours. I wouldn't do long marathon sessions that tire you out unless you have powerful stamina. Shopping is no joke. It's physical, mental, and an emotional sport. The trying on is still movement.

3. SNACKS + MOOD Bring some healthy snacks and water or patronize personal shopping departments that include food so that you can stay in a good mood. These may seem like basics but they do make all the difference. Saks Fifth Avenue, for example, has a menu for its personal shopping clients and have things like healthy salads, nuts, and cheese which can be a godsend.

4. SHOP AT NON-BUSY TIMES When the stores first open on a non-sale weekday is a great time to shop to avoid the crowds.

5. SEASONAL TIMING

   When to shop during the year?

   In North America, fall merchandise starts to arrive in July and August, and spring arrives in January and February. I advise my clients to shop earlier in the season rather than later for the best selection of merchandise. Especially if you are a hard to find size. If you are just graze shopping, meaning you don't have specific needs, then you can shop sales. But generally the really good merchandise and special pieces go first. When I visit off price stores, I can always tell that the merchandise didn't sell somewhere else because the quality is inferior or there is something slightly off. You want the best. Not the second best. Second best items will not get worn and will take up space in your closet.

6. LASER FOCUS Should you shop for your Palm Beach home only in Florida stores? Should you shop for your New York pied-à-terre only in NYC? Should you shop for Aspen when you're in Colorado? Not necessarily. But having an open mind and also, at the same time, laser focusing to what you need is going to help you tremendously. Build your main residence's current season wardrobe first and then move on to your secondary homes. Don't try to shop for all homes at once. It's too much, too fast, and a shortcut

to insanity. If one home is in dire need of being properly stocked you might want to start with that one. Department stores are designed to distract you from your primary goal. That's their job. They want you to get distracted and buy more than you planned to. So it's important you remain laser focused when you shop. Scan the floor. See how it's laid out. Check the map and decide what floors you will look at. Most department stores are organized by designers, and they group designers together based on price point and demographic. So for example, in Saks Fifth Avenue NYC, there is the highest price point floor which houses the personal shopping department (strategically placed) and designers like Azadeline Alaia and Carolina Herrera. It is geared towards the more mature richer client. Then the middle group is geared towards middle priced stock brands like Ralph Lauren, Donna Karan and Issey Miyake. The lower price point floor is geared towards a younger maybe 20-year-old client. They stock designers like Rebecca Taylor, Diane Von Furstenberg, and Alice and Olivia. Once you have your budget you can choose which floors to spend time on. I would suggest skipping any floors where the price points are out of budget for you. Don't torture yourself. Laser focus should also pertain to specific garments. So if you are looking for a dress, don't get distracted by a t-shirt. If you know you need certain colors and cuts don't veer off from this plan. Before you shop, consult your wardrobe master plan and style shopping lists. Make sure you're clear on what you need for each house and potential upcoming event. It also helps to visualize what you would like the garment to look like. Is it form fitting or loose, what vibe should it have, what sort of neckline, and how long should it be? What colors look amazing on you? Don't get too hung up on your style dreams because, sometimes, you don't find what you are looking for exactly and that's okay. Next season is always around the corner.

Certain designers use specific color palettes that work for specific places in the world. For example: Lily Pulitzer-Palm Beach, Bermuda-Pastel and bright colors great for cool skin blonds.

Trina Turk-Miami, Palm Beach, Southern California, Palm Springs-bold prints are good for bright winters with big contrast between hair and skin. Donna Karan-New York City and global travel.

Brunello Cucinelli-Hamptons -muddy muted warm colors great for light autumns and light summers.

7. PULL WIDE Divide your shopping time into 4 sections.
   ~ Pull time
   ~ Try on time
   ~ Decision time
   ~ Check out time

   Pull time means the time when you will walk around the floor and 'pull' items from the floor. It is industry speak for take it off the rack. Some stores may even facilitate this by providing a rolling rack for you to bring along as you pull items. You want to pull way more than you need. Cast a wide net. Try things you may not have looked at before. Some items have hanger appeal and some have body appeal. When you are shopping for a whole new wardrobe follow this strategy. Try on items by category. For example, first try on all the dresses in one chunk of time with shrugs or second layers. Then try on pants, and then try on all the tops. Then pair the winning tops with the winning pants. Discard any pieces that don't go with anything.

8. TRY ON MORE Try on more items than you normally would.

Stretch yourself .

You never know.

If it doesn't work out, no harm no foul.

It might not be a piece for where you are at now but what about your other homes?

I often try on things just to see how it will hang and react to my body .

A good stylist will nudge you to try on new things and know when to back off. As you are trying on, make a maybe or no pile.

9. MAYBE AND NO PILE After the first try on, decide if the item is a contender or if it's a definite NO. No need to make decision quite yet. After you have

tried everything on revisit your maybe pile and review. Ask yourself some questions about the pieces.

~ Do you need this?

~ Is it going to work with the other things in your closet?

~ Will it work for the event you need it for?

~ Can you wear it multiple times?

~ How does the price feel to you?

~ Does it feel worth it?

~ I often add up the maybe purchases and see where you are budget wise.

~ Don't forget that most likely if you work with a personal shopper or personal stylist they will negotiate a special coupon for you, so you will save some money. Especially at stores like Lord and Taylor, who are generous with coupons and sales.

~ You may have to try on an item a second time to get a real answer for yourself. Often the reaction in your face will tell you if you love it or not. It should feel like joy when it's on your body.

10. FEELING FAT DRESS You would think that a personal stylist would ALWAYS feel stylish and would never be challenged by what to wear, right? WRONG. Last Saturday I had my monthly visitor and was feeling a bit bloated. And it was snowing! Totally normal, I know. I was scheduled to attend a dinner party with powerful and fabulous women. I saw it as a fun event but also recognized the potential

for new clients and client referrals. I knew I had to put my best stylish foot forward, but I was having trouble selecting a dress to wear. I realized that my pooch (although completely normal) was throwing me off base. Luckily, I had a dress that I had recently purchased and had not yet gotten tailored. I put it on, and it hid all hints of a pooch. I layered on accessories, a big fur coat, killer boots, and was out the door. Despite feeling not-so-hot internally and contemplating canceling on my friend, my outfit was able to elevate my mood. The evening turned out to be an absolute delight. I made two new friends and got a few compliments on my outfit, and overall the night made me feel SO much better. I've been thinking about that dress, and how as a woman, it's necessary to have my what I call a "I'm feeling fat" dress.

Do you have the occasional day when you're feeling bloated or fat? From your period, from a big meal, from the holidays, from life? Often this "feeling fat" isn't a physical reality but is probably due to small five-pound weight fluctuations that are 100% normal (and, by the way, that other people don't see). The idea that we will all stay the EXACT same weight ALL of the time is destructive thinking. I invite you to anticipate and embrace change in your body. All of my clients know what they have on their list at all times so they can keep an eye out for those items. We all need an arsenal of outfits, and part of that wardrobe should allow for changes in our bodies. So in your closet you should have what I call "feeling fat" dress. It's a dress that makes you look and feel fabulous and it hides any lumps and bumps going on and is maybe slightly bigger than your other dresses. This way you know it will fit and you can attend the event with no issue. You should have a winter and summer version.

Just as I teach my private clients of all sizes, I invite you to shop for that one dress that will give you a bit of leeway in the middle and help you get out the door when you're feeling only 60% hot. One key is to look for a dress in a slimming color such as navy, brown, gray, or an interesting print. Look for details like belly cross draping, and wrap features that help conceal a little belly. Or, try an energizing color that elevates your mood and flatters your features. No matter what details your "feeling fat" look has, make sure the outfit makes you feel absolutely beautiful!

11. GET HELP How to speak a personal shopper's language.

In the big department stores when I bring a client in I use the personal shopping department to be my liaison. Often after I've scoured the store and I cannot locate a certain item I will ask the personal shopper to help. I give her as much specifics as possible. So, for example, instead of saying "I need something to go over this dress," I might say, "I'm looking for a shrug that ends right under the bust in bright colors, price point under $300, in a size 8." That way she can be set up for success or plainly let me know they don't have the item. If they don't have the item, add it to your style shopping list in as much detail as possible and then search online.

12. ONLINE SEARCHING STRATEGIES Use the search functionality on the websites and ability to filter the results. More online shopping resources are in the back of the book for you. I did a whole video on how to maximize online shopping. You can see it at AlexandrAStylist.com/how-to-shop-online.

WHAT STOPS YOU FROM SHOPPING SUCCESS

Maybe you had a meltdown in a store or dressing room before.

A negative memory of shopping as a teenager?

Maybe a color you just hate and brings up bad memories?

Frustration that you can't find what you are looking for so you just buy things out of exasperation?

Or you had a bad day so you buy some things to make you feel better.

But when you get them home the high is gone?

There are so many shopping style blocks, but one of the most common ones is rushing through shopping without being conscious of what you need and are purchasing. It's easy to teach you tactical moves to make shopping easier but harder to cure you of any emotional style blocks standing in your way. I bring this up A LOT, because I find that it is style blocks that are often the thing that prevent a client from making progress the most. Logistics is easy but emotions make it more complicated.

Filling an Emotional Void

During the first few months of working together Anne shared with me, as we were editing her New York closet by the rack, she had a realization. She was remembering pieces and the occasion when she was purchasing them and realizing that a lot of pieces she was buying to 'fill a void' in her emotionally or feeling the pressure to buy something for an event. It was fast and almost harried. There wasn't a moment of calm consciousness where the purchase felt right. She was disconnected. But now in the practice of weeding things out one by one she was learning about herself and how she might slow down.

Some tips to avoid a shopping hangover:

~ Slow down.
~ Relax.
~ Breathe.
~ Ask yourself why are you buying this item? To fill an emotional void, or is it an actual winner?
~ Put something on hold and sleep on it.

Fear and Shopping Don't Mix

What visual message are you sending? While in the closet of a Californian client, I found a couple of outfits that she was a bit prickly about. Without trying them on, she announced that they were 'heatwave' outfits and were badly needed in case of very hot weather. To me, these "heat wave outfits" looked like foreign transactions gone bad. When I had her try them on, we could both see that neither outfit was doing her any favors.

Having a neutral partner (like me) is key in order to take photographs to help you compare exactly what image you project to the one you think you project. During the editing process, we discovered other attractive "heat wave" options, and she was happy to donate the ones that weren't actually serving her needs. During the exchange, I realized that her outfits had been fear purchases. How often do we buy something in panic mode without checking to see if it's really going to be flattering on us? What about when we buy a dress in a rush because we need it for a certain occasion but have no time to properly shop? I see how fear and procrastination can be detrimental to our wardrobes and to our wallets. So, I ask you to filter your purchases through this mental checklist:

~ Does the color flatter my face?
~ Does the shape accentuate the best aspects of my figure?
~ Is it the right message or identity for my life?
~ Will I wear it more than five times
~ Is the price right for my budget?

Have high standards for your image, and you will always be delighted with the outcome. Be patient that the right piece will come along, and it always will. We all feel that gut instinct when we happen across the perfect dress, jacket, or top. Instead of listening to the fear when you shop, listen to that helpful intuition.

You've learned how to maximize your shopping and what can prevent us from success in this area. Now on to some of the common questions I get asked.

COMMON QUESTIONS
What Kinds of Fabrics Should My Garment Be Made of?

Fabric content is a huge factor today, especially with care. Since you travel and move around a lot, I would suggest paying attention to which fabrics breathe, travel well and don't wrinkle. Up in Northeast Harbor Maine where my grandmother summers, there really isn't a good dry cleaner so having items that can be washed or hand washed is key. Finding 100% cotton has become more and more rare these days. It's still possible but not easy because the price of cotton has gone up dramatically. Designers are using more polyester /nylon/ acetate blends. Generally polyester is not a great fabric because it doesn't breathe, holds sweat stains, and can be dry clean only.

Good fabrics for ease of care + comfort = stretch wool, cotton, silk, cashmere, linen/cotton blend

Bad fabrics for ease of care + comfort = polyester, acetate

Thanks to the Laundress, most garments that say dry clean only can be hand washed with their products. I've been testing this faithfully.

So when you are shopping, look at fabric content labels so that you know if caring for the garment will be realistic for you. Bookmark this grid by the Laundress so that you know which ones you can hand wash.

You can opt out of garments because of their fabric content.

Should I Shop in H&M, Gucci, or Haute Couture?

Fast fashion is becoming an environmental crisis. Fast fashion brands like H&M, COS, Old Navy, and Zara produce cheap garments and want you to buy, buy, buy, and then throw them away. The quality is lacking and often they fall apart very quickly. They are constantly shipping new garments to the store, so that you return often and shop often.

Fast fashion is for sure using sweat labor, slave labor, overseas labor, and child labor.

They entice you with hard to believe cheap prices, so in your mind you're thinking, "Well if I don't like it, I haven't wasted much money."

But it is this mentality that is causing such an environmental crisis.

Even if you donate your discarded clothing, only about 15% are usable and the rest get tossed or sold overseas.

From this point forward, I want you to strive to love and wear 80% of your closets and not the standard 20%.

This won't be easy to become a conscious shopper and there is a learning curve, but it's possible.

So from now on, I would like you to buy the best you can afford, love it and wear it.

Focus on quality fabrics, quality construction.

Having less is easier to manage.

If you want to continue to shop fast fashion, please buy only what you know you are going to wear like for t-shirt or pajama basics.

Designers sell expensive clothing usually in two season releases a year, and the price point is higher. The quality is generally higher, and the garment construction is better. Some labels even produce their garments in New York. Some designer clothing may have handmade touches to the garments. Haute Couture is custom clothing made by hand custom fit to your body. Juicy Couture has nothing couture about it!

Generally to be considered Haute Couturier you have to be certified by the Chambre Syndicale de la Haute Couture in France. Therefore, most couturiers are in France. The one exemption in America is Chado, Ralph Rucci who has shown in Paris and has been certified. If you see his garments up close, it is clear the hundreds of hours spent per garment to construct them.

So far we've been talking about clothing, but who doesn't love to shop for shoes.

SHOE SHOPPING

Gorgeous but uncomfortable shoes overfill my client's closets when I meet them. It's the most common style challenge; women own so many pairs of shoes, but only a few comfortable ones get worn and the uncomfortable ones stay home. Most shoe designers are men but I'm hoping to see big change in this industry. Already I'm seeing more and more companies using technology to customize and innovate. True Gault, for example, just launched their iPhone app which allows any woman anywhere in the world to scan her feet, select her shoes, preferred heel height, and color - and they are made for her in just a few weeks in Spain with high quality leathers. A great solution for the working woman who needs to look polished and dressy in heels and still run or walk in comfort. Many of my clients are enjoying their new True Gaults. Feetz is a casual shoes company using 3D printers to make custom shoes. Stay tuned for more advancement in this area.

Working with a Stylist

If after reading this chapter you know that mastering shopping is not something you want to add to your wheelhouse, you can always hire a stylist to shop for you. You might not have the time to dedicate to the hunt for the perfect outfit. You might not want to shop. You might, as my client Kim says, 'love beautiful clothing but hate shopping' and know that won't change soon.

Ellen shared before hiring me that her dream come true was to hand her credit card to a friend who would then shop for her. So walking into a dressing room, prepared just for her, is exactly what she needed to look good for her full life with a successful career in finance, and as a wife and mother of 3. Most of my clients prefer for me to shop for them because it saves them time and money, and they get to try on new styles they would not have picked out for themselves. They enjoy being stretched a little bit out of their style comfort zone and love the compliments that ensue. It's an easy button for them.

Reasons why you may want to hire an independent personal stylist (not to be confused with a department store personal shopper):

- ~ saves time when shopping since you can walk into a fully stocked dressing room curated for you
- ~ saves money (no longer purchase items you won't wear)
- ~ helps you stick to a budget
- ~ you avoid shopping your blind spots
- ~ your stylist will keep track of what you have in your closets and what you have purchased
- ~ preferential treatment is negotiated on your behalf
- ~ easier and stress-free
- ~ stylist will keep you on track with your style goals
- ~ stylist won't let you purchase items that don't flatter your body
- ~ stylist's opinions of items are unbiased and not based on how much you spend
- ~ help finishing outfits that need completion in your wardrobes
- ~ no need to wander the store feeling lost
- ~ don't have to understand or decode current vanity sizing

So whether you can find shopping nirvana yourself or find an ally who can help you solve your style challenges, you can get your multiple closets under control.

CHAPTER **8**

STYLE

Style is the last step of the style prescription process. When I say style I mean the act of styling the pieces together. Basically, trying things on and experimenting. Playing dress-up!!

Once you have finished your shopping trips for this season you want to style it all together in your closet. That means try on new outfit combinations with accessories and document them for reference by taking photos on your phone. You might want to do a series of outfits each for a different home, and then after the outfits are created, send them down to that home. We did this for Anne and her Palm Beach home. She knew she would only be in Palm Beach for a few days at a time, but she was very social down there. We knew when she was there she needed complete outfits that would wow and were complete with the perfect accessories. So, we created a season of outfits fully accessorized, and then they got shipped down to Palm Beach. We made sure to create outfits for all sorts of occasions that she might have coming up. For example, tooling down Worth Avenue, lunch at the club, dinner dates, and benefits were some of the occasions. Once we created the outfits by having her try them on and accessorizing them to perfection, we took photos of the outfits for a folder in her iPad called PALM BEACH, and then sent the whole rack including shoes and accessories down there, completely created. Sometimes in the styling process you will try on a combination and it won't feel 100% right, so we keep mixing and matching till we hit perfection. Then we take the photograph for your reference. Because styling is personalized to the individual, it would be wrong to act like this is teachable. Nevertheless, I'm going to share with you my approach to styling, a few tips, and hope it helps make it easier for you.

I practice the art of very simple styling. The first thing to learn is how to mix and match, or just match. Here are a few approaches to try.

Go Monochrome

Pair like color items together, and then add the same color shoes and metallic purse.

Keep It Balanced

Pair a looser item with a tighter item. Balance a voluminous piece with a more form fitting piece.

Complementary Colors

Pair complementary colors together. For example, a tan top with chocolate pants.

Build Around a Star Piece

Start with a star piece that has lots of personality like a print or embellished, and then add a basic that balances the piece. Add one more piece of flair in an accessory but more simple.

Let's say you have a print top. What would you wear on the bottom? Find a color within the print that flatters you and wear that on the bottom following the balance rules of one tighter and one looser as above.

Stay in Season

Style the clothing with pieces of the same season. Don't pair a sleeveless silk blouse with tiny holes in it with a heavy wool pant. It will just look odd.

Have an Order

Proceeding with an order in which you put on the items, can help the process tremendously.

Start with the key piece you want to wear for day.

~ Undergarments
~ Dress
~ Shoes and stockings - same color or neutral-like nude or black or brown
~ Necklace

- ~ Earrings
- ~ Ring
- ~ Bag
- ~ Coat
- ~ Scarf
- ~ Hat

Or

- ~ Undergarments
- ~ Printed Pants
- ~ Top in a color from the printed pants
- ~ Belt
- ~ Shoes
- ~ Necklace
- ~ Earrings
- ~ Ring
- ~ Coat
- ~ Scarf
- ~ Hat
- ~ Bag

Try to stick to 3 colors or less. Because simple is easier, and no one wants complicated.

ACCESSORIES

When adding accessories, I simply recommend wearing monochromatic looks with one new pop of color introduced. So in hot weather, all white with a splash of red or pink. In cold weather, all gray with one blue scarf. Having color and accessory wardrobes at multiple houses could be complicated or it can be simple. To simplify, limit your color palettes.

There is one big decision you need to make for yourself. Are you going to stock each house with its own accessories, or are you going to use the same ones at each house? There are certain shoes and bags that very much work in certain places, like a wicker bag works in places like Nantucket but wouldn't work in New York. A very sparkly Judith Leiber minaudiere works very much in Florida, and some can work in New York. And then some purses work everywhere. So I guess it depends on what kinds of pieces you have and what you want to have. Would you rather have 5 bags that only go with 1 outfit, or 1 bag that goes with most of your outfits? Again, it's back to if you are a chameleon or more of a uniform basic dresser.

In the accessory department, if you want to keep things simple just purchase metallic accessories like shoes and bags, and stop trying to match exact colors. Metallics act like neutrals but are more interesting and give another dimension to your look. They are also very easy to mix too. Mixed metallic shoes are like gold in my books because pulling on one of the other metallic shades becomes so easy. Basic black is also a very common way to go with all your accessories. It's safe, but I don't always recommend it.

How to Be Chic When You Want to Wear Sweats Every Day

I spent some time working with clients throughout Marin County and San Francisco and have witnessed firsthand what the biggest style challenges are in the region, and have some great solutions. It seems to me that, due to California's healthy and active gym lifestyle, most women are living their lives primarily in their Lululemon - upscale sweats.

As a personal style expert, and based on some interactions with several Marin women, I've realized that there is a lack of knowledge about what could be the next step up style-wise. They wonder, "How can I get out of my active wear, but still be super comfortable and look more polished?"

The answer is really about balancing the casual with the dressy. Here are two outfit ideas:

1. Your best fitting, most stylish dark sweats or leggings (no baggy butts, please)
   ~ a stylish jacket or sweater
   ~ jewelry
   ~ dressier leather sneakers (navy or metallic are great)
   ~ scarf
2. Your dressiest dark wash tailored jean
   ~ navy cotton stretchy jacket with tailored touches
   ~ jewelry
   ~ black booties
   ~ optional scarf

Styling for normal day to day life is one thing, but what happens when you get hurled a curveball? A last minute invitation to a formal event? What to do?

Secret to Last Minute Invitations

If your best friend invited you last minute to a wedding in Vermont in the summer but it was only 50 degrees, would you be able to quickly dress and feel amazing in your outfit? My clients are able to handle any curveball that is thrown out at them because together we have created a style look book with outfits that have already been created and tried on.

This method takes longer and is more work than just taking photographs of the garments flat, and mixing and matching, but it is MUCH more effective because you have seen the outfit on your body and have felt how it FEELS. (I have found that something matched together on a bed does not always translate well on the body.)

In our styling sessions, we also walk through all sorts of scenarios that might arise and make you freak out. By planning outfits in advance it sets you up for success.

Some scenarios that are common:

~ Black tie event but you don't want to wear a gown
~ Black tie event where you know every woman is going to wear a strapless gown but you would like to be warm and not freezing in the ballroom that is kept at sub temps.
~ Masked ball
~ Halloween party with a theme

~   Themed birthday party
~   Holiday parties

So, the secret to getting dressed in a flash and feeling confident is preparation and having me as a partner makes the journey all that much easier.

The styling step is where your personality has a chance to shine.

How you put things together is what makes you unique.

So have fun with it.

Play around, experiment till you get that feel of perfection in the mirror.

HOW TO REMEMBER YOUR LOOKS

We are all busy.

It's a fact.

Life is fast.

So many of my clients do not want to spend hours thinking about what they are going to wear. After going through my intensive Style package they are set, because they have a look book made just for them with looks for each season and for each house. Since I'm taking you through all the steps they go through, you can, too. You can take the photos that you took during your style sessions and make them into iPhoto look books, or you can easily just store them in a special folder on your iPhone or make a Pinterest board. In your phone you can even divide them into folders like casual looks, work looks, dressy looks, black tie looks. Or you can organize them by house and then by seasons. For example, Palm Beach - black tie, Palm Beach - casual lunch, New York - work, New York - dressy events. Whichever way works best for you and is easiest to access.

Here's how I organize the books that I make for my clients.

One book for Fall/Winter and one book for Spring/Summer. If you live in a place where there is very little difference in seasons like California you can just make one book. And include some rain looks and ski trip looks.

I start the book with casual looks, then showcase work looks, and end with special occasion wear.

I make sure to shoot complete looks with accessories and close ups of jewelry for later reference.

Only shoot outfits that make your heart sing.

There will be outfits that you play around with and then you decide aren't good enough.

That's okay.

No need to shoot the outfits if they don't feel 100% amazing.

If you can shoot in daylight that is best, and get head to toe to include shoes. This process takes longer than shooting items flat, but it's so much more effective than shooting random items flat because you don't know how they will really work together on the body.

Check out the resource part of the book for some apps that will help you with cataloguing your wardrobes. You might choose to use a style app to catalogue your looks and to digitally create new looks. This is entirely up to you. If it sounds like fun, try it out. If not, no big deal.

Or hire someone to do the initial work of photographing all your pieces.

Creating outfits and at least photographing them will help you in those moments when you feel you have nothing to wear. You can simply flip through your iPhone or book or app, and peruse your outfit choices based on weather and what you are wanting to wear that day.

We've finished going through the style prescription process, which means you now have all the tools you need to get started. The next few chapters are going to cover how to care for your items, get them to your multiple homes, and give you tips about what to wear during what kind of weather, as well as tips by location.

CHAPTER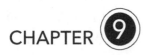

GARMENT CARE

With multiple homes, garment care can become more of a crucial issue. Let's say you leave some cashmere sweaters in your Maine home uncleaned for eight months. For sure when you return there will be moth holes if not cleaned and stored properly.

I remember my grandmother bemoaning Maine because there was no good dry cleaner in town to trust. So, her solution was to bring her dry cleaning back to Connecticut after the season.

Not the best solution, but it was before the Laundress products were born.

In this chapter, I'm going to share with you my top tips and products for garment care, so that you can care for the new items you love to wear. With proper care, they will last so much longer and it is better on the environment.

Ever since I discovered the Laundress products and blog, my life and my clients' lives have been forever changed. You see, I try out everything myself as a customer before recommending any product. I was hating the dry cleaner. I would spend $15 dry cleaning a dress, and it would come back smelling of chemicals and the underarms wouldn't be odor free. Laundress has this handy chart that will show you how to care for all your garments based on fabric content.

So many items that are labeled dry clean only can in fact be hand washed with their products. I have been starting to hand wash some of my dresses using their delicate wash product, and they come out cleaner and fresher. Don't want to do the hand washing yourself? Hire it out to your housekeeper or hire a service. Some items you can put in a mesh bag and use delicate cycle and Laundress products in your washing machine. Just make sure the water temperature is correct. Check the resource section for info on Allo Laverie that focuses on hand washing fine linens. They do pickup and delivery in Manhattan and also do it by mail order service. french-handlaundry.com. You also can hang dry your washed clothes and skip the dryer. It prolongs the life of garments.

Toughest Stains

Sweat stains: Most stains can be removed if you act quickly. I used to think sweat stains were irreversible. With most stains, the longer you let them sit. The harder they are to remove. If you can spray oxy clean or use a stain remover product from the Laundress immediately on sweat stains, they generally come out. For sweat stains that are old, they can be removed but with a combination of bleach alternative and stain remover from the Laundress, and then pour hot water on it and let it sit. Rinse and repeat a few times. This takes a while, but for your favorite items it can be worth it. I revived an over eight year old dress that was not being worn due to sweat stains.

Blood: You're going to hate this advice but it works! Immediately spit on the blood on the garment. This saved my white couch. The proteins in your spit break down the blood very quickly.

Then follow up with Laundress products based on fabric type.

What to Hang and What to Fold

Knits should be folded and not hung in all of your homes. Why? Because they stretch out, otherwise. This includes knit tops, sweaters, knit dresses, knit scarves, knit skirts, etc.

They will stretch out because they're knit from one continuous thread. So how do you know if it's a knit and not a woven? Knits look like a tiny row of braids and a woven looks like a basket weave. The holes in knits are larger too. Crochet items should be folded and not hung, as well.

How to Care for Scarves

Silk scarves can be hand washed in a delicate wash and stored in a canvas box. You may choose to shuttle your scarves between each house because they don't take up much room, or relegate certain scarves for each house. If you have a bright print that feels like Florida or Palm Springs, you may choose to leave it at that house. Leaving thick wool and cashmere scarves at your ski house is also a great idea because they are bulky. Just make sure they are washed before leaving behind and storing.

Sweater Pilling

Sweater pilling is inevitable. Even the finest cashmere pills. You don't have to get angry about it.

Just get a sweater stone from The Laundress. Stay away from the little machine trimmers as they can damage your sweaters. Make sure to de-pill at the end of the season before you leave that house, so that they are fresh at your next visit.

Garment Repair

Before leaving a house for a stretch of time, review your closet and take out anything that needs to be washed or possibly repaired. This means missing buttons, unraveling hem, strap broken, or holes. Simple fixes can usually be handled by a dry cleaner that has a tailor but for more challenging repairs or alterations, seek out a true tailor. Check the resources guide section of this book for more info.

Even if your knits get a hole, they can most likely be repaired by French American Weaving Company or Alter Knit in NYC. Alter Knit does a lovely mail order business in the US. Chicago has Without a Trace. Invisible Mending is in London. There are details in the resources section in the back.

It's good to do a sweep of your closet before you close up a house of everything that should be repaired or fixed so that when you return, it's taken care of.

The better you care for what you have, the longer they will last and the CPW (cost per wear) will reduce. It's much nicer to have less but better stuff, and most small things can be fixed easily.

So don't just throw away a garment because it's missing a button or needs to be hemmed. If your stuff is in good condition, it will be easier to donate or sell the items. Most things that get donated end up in landfills.

WHEN TO TOSS:	WHEN TO DONATE:
~irreparable holes, stains ~worn out bras, underwear, bathing suits, ~socks ~faded or stretched out ~looking super tired	~good condition but no longer needed or wanted ~items that aren't flattering on you ~no longer feels powerful ~gentle used bras to @freethegirls on Instagram or a local bra drive

Garment care is going to matter more to you since you are managing your style in multiple homes. And now that you have nice things that you love, you're going to want them to last. Especially if you are keeping items at homes when you are not there. Make sure your garments are stored clean. Doing a sweep of what needs to be cleaned, fixed, or shaved before you leave a house is a great practice to keep on top of the process.

CHAPTER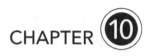

MANAGING, PACKING, AND SHIPPING

D o you want to feel like the same person style wise everywhere in the world?

Or do you want to be more of a chameleon depending on where you are in the world?

Would you wear a Pucci print sundress in St. Barts that you would never wear in NYC?

Or a nautical dress in Nantucket?

My client Anne prefers to define herself style wise by each house. She has decided to go the route of stocking every house with the relevant outfits and travel with the bare minimum between houses, just a few pieces of jewelry to accessorize. And when they travel to Europe, because they travel private, we get her packed with every outfit planned and accessorized. Women like Melinda Gates prefer to be more basic and uniform-like. Every house must have a set of her favorite sunglasses, basic khaki shorts, and classic white crisp shirts. I have worn dresses with my grandparents in Hobe Sound where it's very preppy that I would only wear there. They are dresses for that environment and scene and no other. Maybe they would also work in Nantucket or Northeast Harbor Maine.

In this chapter, you are going to learn about managing your style with ease in each of your homes. And then I will offer some options of how to physically move items from house to house. You will learn the advantages of shipping or traveling with your items, and decide which options work best for your lifestyle.

Is it possible to travel with no luggage today?

With multiple homes and some planning, yes it is.

We have more services these days than ever that make your life easier. Apple apps and services that cater towards multiple homeowner needs. Most of the closet management apps take up a lot of time to set up because you have to document what you have. Obviously having home managers help make your life easier. If you can outsource this, it can be helpful, because with multiple homes and multiple closets, the sheer number of items can be daunting. My grandmother's solution was to shuttle her clothing up and down the east coast in a van with hanging rods installed, driven by one of her staff. I would suggest even if your closets are different in each home that you try to organize them in a similar fashion.

If your underwear are always in the top drawer, put them in the top drawer in every house. If you keep your tops on the left side of the closet, keep them that way in every house. Try to create the ultimate closet in the first home and then model the others after the first. It will keep you from getting discombobulated. This also applies to the kitchen and the bathroom. Create a check in / check out station in every house, so that you never lose your keys.

Having a system will help. Here are some amazing tools to make managing, organizing, and packing a breeze.

Custom Closets

Having a custom built closet is the ultimate luxury. But make sure it's designed with exactly what you have, or choose the ELFA system that is adjustable. Being able to make changes to your closet by season is savvy. ELFA is also much more affordable than a fully custom closet. Bring your measurements into the store, and they will guide you through designing the best closets for you. I designed four closets at a time 9 years ago and am still super happy with the outcome. Installation is easy to delegate, or you can have them install it for you.

Garde Robe- Luxury Storage and Valet Service

This service will photograph and catalogue every garment you send them for a price of $25 an item. This helps if you don't have staff already in place. Then you can order your garments to be shipped to the house of your choice. They also handle the dry cleaning and cleaning of the garments and make sure they are stored properly. This proper storage is crucial for one of a kind and couture garments. So, in a way they handle managing, packing, shipping, and cleaning of your garments. Talk about an easy button!

Style Book App

An iOS app works with iPhone, iPad, and iTouch that helps you manage what you have in your closets digitally.

PROS
~   You can erase the background of the photos
~   Once it's set up you can mix and match new combinations that you might not have thought of
~   You can upload your images into their categories or make up your own categories like main house, beach house, ski house, etc.
~   There is a nice 'packing' feature of the closet and the 'calendar' feature will allow you to assign looks to certain days.

CONS
~   Slight learning curve
~   Can be a lot of upfront work

This iOS app is great for capsule wardrobes, because it's easy to use for small amounts of garments and accessories. But in your case, you will most likely want to get some help because importing and photographing all of your clothing and accessories at all of your homes will be quite a chore. Depending on how many pieces you have. But this is the preferred app if you want to see outfits made together instead of just individual shots of pieces. The other thing to note is that just because they look good together on the screen won't guarantee they will work on your body, depending on how the garments drape and react to each other. I would start with doing this for one of your secondary houses with the least amount of stuff first, and then see how it goes. You can then add for the other residences.

Packing

When I was 16, I went to Oxford, England for a summer program that included Shakespeare and photography. I knew we would also be taking a trip to Paris. I was beyond excited, and being a Virgo and daughter of a Virgo, I wanted to be super prepared and organized. Packing was one of my Mother's forte, and she often prepped for over a month for a trip. I'm not sure where I got the idea, but I got it in my mind that I would create outfits and pack each outfit in a Ziploc bag complete with matching underwear and socks. At the time, I was wearing shorts, skirts, and pants combinations. I was so excited by this packing hack I invented. I was wearing lots of color and fun prints, and it was a great way to get dressed easily every day. It did help especially when I went to Paris, and I still use Ziplock bags for underwear, socks, and toiletries. I have since then simplified my packing for trips and life, and generally only wear dresses or pants. It makes my life easier.

Folding

I would never win an award for folding since I never worked in retail, but reading Marie Kondo's book changed the way I fold and store my clothing. Her idea of folding garments into smaller rectangles and then organizing like a file folder so that you can see everything from above is brilliant. Stacking folded shirts in a drawer means you never get to the bottom shirt and is inefficient.

Packing Cubes

I learned about packing cubes from my nomadic friend in Mallorca. She was traveling the world with a backpack and mostly via yacht and swore by her packing cubes. They are the same concept as my Ziploc bags, but they are more environmental, durable, and breathable. First, you fold the item flat, and then you roll it and insert into the packing cube. They condense your stuff, so you can often fit more into your suitcase than if you just placed them in there. The advantage is having a nice sorting system so that you can find exactly what you need, which if you are moving around a lot this can be helpful. Once you arrive you don't even need much room in a drawer and unpacking is faster, since you're just taking out your cubes and they are already sorted.

Space Bags

I love these for condensing items and then storing them. Let's say you have lots of bulky sweaters or bedding you need to store and shrink. Voila! Takes up so much less space.

Travel Steamer

The best way to get out wrinkles. I use mine all the time, not just when I am traveling. It's small, easy to store, and easy to bring when you travel. In a pinch, you can hang your garment in your bathroom as you take a hot shower for a quick no fuss steam. Steam the garment from the inside of the garment, and make sure all the water sputters out before starting to steam. You don't want the canister too full. My top travel steamer choice is included in my second book Vetted by a Stylist.

Luggage Forward

Luggage Forward is a wonderful service that ships your suitcases and oversized items like golf clubs, skis, and bicycles. No need to transfer your clothing to boxes; they ship in your luggage, and you can order it all from your smartphone or tablet. Pricing is transparent and is cheaper if you allow longer ship time. Each bag automatically is insured for $500.

DIY

Just plain old FedEx, UPS, or post office. This winter I'm spending two months in Florida writing this book and serving clients. I brought two small bags with about 2 weeks' worth of clothing, as I like to pair down and go minimalist. I knew I would need dressy outfits for one short portion of my trip, so I shipped 4 dresses and shoes to that address and when I was done, shipped them back to my NYC address. I also, in advance, made up a box of cold weather outfits for an author conference in Washington, DC that will ship to my hotel and then will get shipped back to NYC after they are worn. I then don't need to return to NYC to get these clothes or have them take up space in my Florida suitcases. I use online resources to print the shipping labels. A pretty affordable solution for a lady on the go. Also, good if you are just shipping a few items.

However, you decide to manage all of your closets, make sure to have a trial period and then reassess. If it doesn't work for you, try another method till you find your groove.

Weather is often a massive roadblock for my clients and their style, so I've included a whole chapter about it up next.

CHAPTER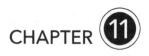

HANDLE TEMPERATURE FLUCTUATIONS LIKE A BOSS

t's hot.

It's cold.

When it comes down to it, weather can stop you from leaving the house. It can add more time and stress into getting dressed. It can cause major overwhelm and confusion. So, I'm here to help you with that style block.

WHAT TO WEAR WHEN YOU ARE AFFECTED BY THE WEATHER?

Freezing at Benefits

Who else here finds benefits held in hotels freezing? My client does and airs her grievances not only about the temperature but also by the popularity contest going on with the outfits. She has no desire to dress like a Barbie version of herself and although sees the value in looking good, doesn't want to become a slave to it. I get it! Some of us naturally run cold, so going strapless black tie in a chilly ballroom is not going to happen. This is an issue that can frankly happen to you at any house, whether it's in New York or Palm Beach, so the key is being prepared.

Here are some solutions to wear:

- ~ Warm tights and then long underwear underneath your long gown
- ~ Dramatic and cropped fur caplet or jacket
- ~ Tuxedo jacket over sleek jumpsuit
- ~ Long sleeve gown
- ~ Long sleeve dressy top and long skirt
- ~ Very dressy embroidered or metallic coat over slim pants (this one is very easy to travel with because this kind of coat/dress can be also worn with jeans)

Summer Wedding Woes

Anne and her husband were invited to a summer wedding in Vermont. Which was fine except for the weather threw a curveball. It was a cold couple of days, and Anne was sensitive to cold. What to wear to a summer wedding in cold weather? Her planned outfit was a light summery dress, and now that wasn't going to cut it! So, she found a Ralph Lauren ensemble including a light mauve coat. A light-colored coat is the perfect solution for chilly summer occasions. The coat, with matching dress and fine jewelry, pulled it off. If you want a summer coat to blend in multiple locations and occasions go for a slightly metallic textured fabric, and it will go with almost any dress.

Chic and Warm While It's Freezing Out

It's snowing like a banshee and you have to look fabulous, but you would rather curl up on the couch and watch old movies. If you live anywhere snowy or spent significant time in a snowy region you should have an arsenal of outfits that are fabulous and cozy.

~ Long underwear to wear under pants. Silk or wool: it's really up to personal preference
~ Super heavy cashmere tights. Make sure to check fabric content
~ Full-length wool dress – I have one from Zaia in Paris that is so warm and cozy
~ Cashmere sweater dress
~ Chic fitted turtleneck paired with a festive necklace or scarf
~ Chic faux fur or real fur vest (make sure it's waist-defining and doesn't add weight in the middle

region). One of my favorites is by Patrizia Luca, which is rabbit fur and very reasonably priced

~ Show-stoppingly fabulous vintage fur coat to make an entrance to that party when it's 10 degrees. Mine belonged to my Mother, and it practically stops traffic and keeps me toasty

~ Chic hooded layer

~ A furry trapper hat that covers the ears. My top pick is Furtzane Faux Fur Hat

~ Full-length hooded down coat with waist definition and down content of 550+ (Make sure the hood fits snug or it won't keep you warm.) Postcard, Via Spiga, and Canada Goose make great ones

~ Really warm socks like cashmere or wool

~ Waterproof boots with fuzzy wool lining – My Timberlands aren't lined yet work well for me, but note that plastic Wellies and Hunter boots will never keep you warm. And Zappos pays shipping both ways

~ Gloves with either cashmere or fur lining. Sorry, PETA, but fur really keeps you warm. Also, hand warmers really help

~ You lose so much of your heat through your head. If you bundle your head, neck, and feet, that's a great foundation for keeping warm

~ IGNORE earmuffs, headbands, and hats that don't cover your ears. They will do nothing for you in extreme weather

Looking Polished When It's Sweltering Out

With over 100 degree temperatures in NYC, the clothing-optional water junkies at Harbin are sounding kinda smart right about now. Thought I would share my staying cool and looking cool tips with you: Synthetics don't breathe, which is bad news this year because cotton has often been replaced by poly and rayon blends. Cotton used to be cheap and plentiful, but due to the skyrocketing costs, designers have been sourcing other fabric blends. Read your labels carefully if you want to stay cool. I've created a video for you about how to stay cool and stylish when it's hot out. You can watch at AlexandrAStylist.com/how-to-stay-cool-this-summer.

Fabrics that Breathe:
~ Cotton
~ Tencel blend
~ Linen
~ Light wool

Cuts:
~ Having room under the arms is key
~ Sleeveless
~ Long maxi dresses on the loose side
~ Flowing cuts that provide less contact with fabric to skin

ADDITIONAL TIPS
~ Wear a big hat to keep the sun off your face

~ Mott-50, Cabana Life, and Coolibar make sun protective clothing

~ I take a strip of cotton from an old shirt, soak in ice water, and wear around my neck.

~ I got the idea when I tried a neck bandoo on a trip to Greece

~ In extreme cases, I carry a stylish umbrella, and it makes a big difference in temperature

~ Drink hot beverages like tea, which help cool you down even more. This sounds counter-intuitive, but it works

~ I get cold in all the AC buildings so I layer with a scarf, shawl, or cardigan with easy air flow

~ I recently picked up this open weave wrap from Anthropologie that has great ventilation and is stylish

So, no matter what temperature roadblocks get thrown your way, hopefully, you feel more prepared. I check the weather frequently on my phone and make sure to consult 'real feel' temperature before deciding what to wear. In this case, knowledge is power and bonus points for creativity.

CHAPTER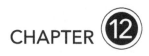

CITY-BASED STYLE

Most all of us travel these days. In fact, I have yet to meet a person that doesn't say, "I love to travel." But each spot is so different style-wise, and I've found that often clients would ask me what to wear in certain hotspots in the world. Because of that, I decided to include this quick guide so that you can get some inspiration of what to wear.

Here are some ideas of what to wear when you visit these hot spots.

Miami, Florida
~ Shorter, sexier, brighter, metallic, designer brands
~ Flashy to the max
~ Designer who captures the spirit: Roberto Cavalli
~ Instagram for inspiration: @emiliopucci

Palm Beach, Florida
~ Bright sunny colors and pastels
~ Playful prints and lots of jewelry
~ If you've got it flash it here
~ Dolce & Gabbana
~ @foggoffashion

Hobe Sound, Florida
~ More understated than and preppy than Palm Beach
~ Make sure your hemlines aren't too short but still wear fun colors
~ Lily Pulitzer
~ @advancedstyle

Northeast Harbor, Maine
~ Shabby chic reigns here
~ The wealthy do not flaunt it here at all
~ Slightly nautical works here, too
~ Patagonia, J. Crew
~ @katenorthrup

Boston, Massachusetts
~ Preppy and a bit international chic
~ Boss
~ @nicholeotchy

New York, Upper East Side
~ Classy, preppy, chicest of chic
~ The more polished and expensive the better

~ Fine jewelry only
~ Chanel
~ @blaireadiebee

Meatpacking
~ Flashy and chic. Shorter hemlines work
~ Black reigns.
~ Diane Von Furstenberg

Williamsburg, Brooklyn
~ Hipster heaven
~ Artsy and weird works here
~ All Saints
~ @michellejoni

St. Barts
~ Much like Florida but classier with a bit more taste
~ Calypso
~ @mersur

Nantucket
~ Nautical and preppy
~ Ralph Lauren
~ @hilaryrushford

Santa Monica, LA
~ Seaside casual and breezy
~ James Pearse
~ @lindsayalbanese

Palm Springs, CA
~ Brights and 60's mod
~ Trina Turk
~ @trinaturk

San Francisco, CA
~ Business casual but still polished
~ Elie Tahari

Aspen, CO
~ Apres ski cozy. Bring your most expensive and flashy ski outfits
~ Loro Piana

Marin County
~ Khaki casual
~ Yoga wear all the time is perfectly acceptable
~ But your car better be luxury
~ LuluLemon

Paris, France
~ Ultra chic with an Avant guard twist
~ Artistic works here too
~ YSL
~ @meganhess_official

Hamptons
~ Dressy and chic or casual and cozy
~ Breezy colors

~ Brunello Cucinelli
~ @arianarockefeller

CHAPTER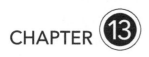

WRAPPING UP

Thank you so much for coming on this journey with me, and I hope you found this book helpful in your quest to stay stylish in all of your homes. When I'm quiet and think about why I do this work, I realize that I do it for the love. Being able to change another woman's life so dramatically fills my heart with love, and I'm grateful to have been a catalyst in something bigger. All of my clients come to me about their closets, but what they don't often realize is that their desire for a style upgrade is a result of another major change in their life.

Because all of my client's situations are so much more layered than having issues with their style, they are often amidst great change in their life. No two are alike.

~ Some are getting promoted or running their own companies

~ Some are getting divorced

~ Some have lost major weight

~ Some are getting their health in order

~ Some are adjusting to a new life and new marriage

~ Some are dealing with children growing up

~ So many are juggling life in multiple places and traveling a lot

And I get to help them through major transformations, look and feel better, and emerge a transformed woman.

Confident.

Powerful.

Prepared.

And ready for anything.

Bridget, a very kind client who splits her time between Manhattan and Upstate New York, recovering from cancer, reclaiming her body and style, said to me after working together, "Every woman should get to feel this way."

I hope that this book has given you the tools you need to infuse your hectic life with a style that supports you. Now it's time for you to decide whether you are going to take this information and apply it yourself, or if you are going to get help and support.

My wish is that you find the right path for you and that your closets become a place of serenity and support.

RESOURCES

ONLINE SHOPPING

A note on the landscape of retail:

What has changed in the past 5-10 years in 'fashion' is that luxury has become obtainable for the masses and is no longer an elite club. Quality has deteriorated. Simple, well-made clothing in great fabrics have become challenging to find. More and more designers have moved in on the 20 year olds' market and size 2 market. Fast fashion dominates the field. Petites and plus size sections in stores have been reduced or eliminated. They do exist online, but this is often the hardest size to fit. In my professional opinion, shopping has become harder and more challenging even though we have more choices than ever. Here are my top online spots to shop:

~ Zappos
~ Nordstrom
~ Macys
~ Bergdorf Goodman
~ Colette.fr - very trendy and young perspective

~ Anthropologie-has nice petites expanded section now
~ Trina Turk
~ Elie Tahari - also check their selection at department stores because they stock different items at each
~ Net-a-porter
~ Moda Operandi
~ Lord and Taylor - in person over online
~ Charm and Chain

BRAS AND UNDERGARMENTS
~ Linda's - specialize in larger sizes
~ Lulalu - small sizes
~ Eve's Apple's Lingerie - small sizes
~ True and Co - online bra fitting
~ ThirdLove - bras in half sizes
~ Instagram.com@freethegirls - bra donation service

SERVICES TO MAKE YOUR LIFE EASIER
~ Quintessentially
~ Mahler Private Staffing

KNIT REPAIR
~ Alter Knit - NYC + SHIPS
~ French American Weaving Company - NYC
~ Invisible Mending - Chicago
~ Without a Trace - London

ORGANIZATION
- ~ Container Store
- ~ Muji
- ~ Elfa
- ~ California Closets

APPS
- ~ Style Book
- ~ Instyle what to wear with every color guide

RENTAL SERVICES
- ~ Rent the Runway - occasion dresses + accessories
- ~ Bag Borrow Steal - handbag
- ~ Adorn - high end jewelry
- ~ RocksBox - costume jewelry
- ~ Le Tote - everyday casual wear
- ~ Le Tote - maternity wear

MAIL ORDER STYLE BOXES
- ~ Cake Style
- ~ Stitch fix
- ~ Box of Style by Rachel Zoe
- ~ Goodebox
- ~ Green Beauty box

MULTI USE GARMENTS
- ~ Encircled
- ~ Jia Collection
- ~ Ioanna Kourbella

~ Coolibar shawl top

ONLINE CONSIGNMENT
~ The Real Real
~ Material WRLD
~ ThredUp
~ Portero
~ Crown and Caliber

SELL YOUR CLOTHING – SAME DAY CASH
~ Beacon's Closet - NYC
~ Buffalo Exchange - NYC

STORAGE
~ The Vault in London
~ Garde Robe
~ The Box Butler
~ Make Space
~ Luggage Forward

SUN PROTECTION
~ Coolibar
~ Mott-50
~ Cabana Life
~ Devita Solar mineral sunscreen moisturizer

TRAVEL ESSENTIALS
~ Sholdit

ACKNOWLEDGEMENTS

Special Thanks to:

Nina Roy

GMP + GFC

Sandra Gault

Susan Blake

Angela Lauria

Cynthia Kane

Nikki Groom

Michelle Rodriguez

Lisa Colletti

Yvonne Grand

Kim Orcutt

Susan Plumeri

Donna Chazen

Ronda Greenawalt

Lisa Rios

Michiko Boorberg

Nadezhda Savinova

Marc Russo

To the Morgan James Publishing team: Special thanks to David Hancock, CEO & Founder for believing in me and my message. To my Author Relations Manager, Gayle West, thanks for making the process seamless and easy. Many more thanks to everyone else, but especially Jim Howard, Bethany Marshall, and Nickcole Watkins.

ABOUT THE AUTHOR

Alexandra Suzanne Greenawalt is a Manhattan-based personal stylist, author, and speaker. She has written two previous books-Secrets of a Fashion Stylist and *Vetted by a Stylist.* Her photoshoot fashion styling work has been published in *Japanese Vogue, The New York Times, InStyle Magazine, Marie Claire Magazine, Surface Magazine*, and many more.

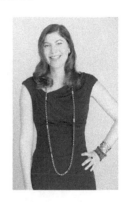

Alexandra has been a guest style expert at several media outlets including Wake Up with Al on the Weather Channel, CNN Money, Yahoo Finance, Real Simple, Fab Fit Fun, Shoptopia, and Sheknows.

Alexandra has worked with celebrities such as Jennifer Hudson, Christina Ricci, Duran Duran, and Antonia Bennett. Since 2001 she has been a catalyst for women's style transformations. Her signature 1:1 program the Style Re-invention is a top to bottom complete style makeover that creates confidence and ease.

Semi nomadic she works with women all over the globe.

THANK YOU

Thank you so much for reading this book.

As a gift to you, besides the workbook that compliments the book that you can download at AlexandrAStylist.com/workbook.

I'm offering a complimentary video. You will learn whether you have a shopping problem or a styling problem, and what next steps you can take.

Access the video at AlexandrAStylist.com/style-help-video

I work with a select few women all over the globe either over a weekend, a season, or per year.

If you would like a complimentary style assessment session go to AlexandrAStylist.com/style-call

How to contact me directly:

www.alexandrastylist.com
ag@alexandrastylist.com
917-674-8404

I so look forward to connecting with you.

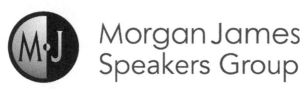

Morgan James
Speakers Group

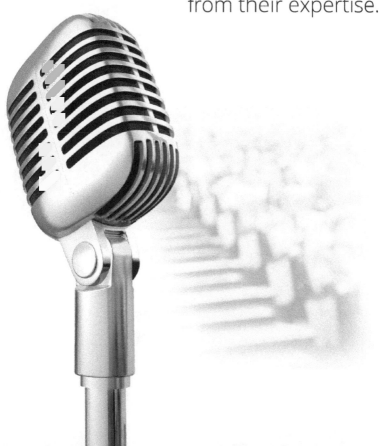

↗ www.TheMorganJamesSpeakersGroup.com

We connect Morgan James published
authors with live and online events
and audiences who will benefit
from their expertise.